NEUROFEEDBACK

FUNCTIONS, APPLICATIONS AND EFFECTS

NEW DEVELOPMENTS IN MEDICAL RESEARCH

Additional books and e-books in this series can be found
on Nova's website under the Series tab.

NEW DEVELOPMENTS IN MEDICAL RESEARCH

NEUROFEEDBACK

FUNCTIONS, APPLICATIONS AND EFFECTS

MICHAEL C. HELLINGER
EDITOR

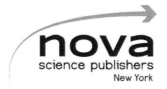

nova
science publishers
New York

NOTICE TO THE READER

Library of Congress Cataloging-in-Publication Data

ISBN: 978-1-53615-167-1

Published by Nova Science Publishers, Inc. † New York

CONTENTS

PREFACE

Neurofeedback: Functions, Applications and Effects presents a number of possible applications for neurofeedback in offender treatment, including perpetuators of domestic violence and various other forms of violent and anti-social behavior, certain forms of sexually abusive behavior, and criminal behavior of an obsessive–compulsive nature. A global description of this method is presented, followed by a brief overview of the empirical evidence of its efficacy in specific relevant treatment areas.

To accomplish a targeted impact of neurofeedback on specific cortical functions, EEG-based local brain activity neurofeedback training was developed by Bauer et al. (2011). With this approach, an implemented algorithm automatically identifies and localizes EEG-sources in successive sLORETA solutions. Based on this information, the feedback is exclusively controlled by EEG-generating sources within a selected cortical region of training. In order to individually and precisely locate and define the region of training, the use of evoked potentials of known local origin is recommended.

In one study, a total of 30 Iranian veterans with spinal cord injuries were randomly assigned to either neurofeedback, physical training, or a control condition. At the beginning of the study and four weeks later, reaction times and balance were objectively measured. Compared to the control condition over time, reaction times improved in the neurofeedback condition, while balance improved in the physical training condition.

Compared to a conventional treatment condition, neurofeedback and physical training improved skills in specific areas of motor control.

The authors go on investigate the effect of neurofeedback training on the motor performance and conscious motor processing of skilled dart players. The subjects consisted of 20 males. The research was conducted in five phases, including: pre-test, training neurofeedback, posttest 1, under pressure test and posttest 2.

Additionally, the authors investigate the effect of one session of neurofeedback training on the motor performance of elite and non-elite volleyball players. The research was conducted in three phases: pre-test, training neurofeedback, and post-test.

The effect of Quiet Mind Training on alpha power and dart throwing is also studied. A total of 20 novice dart players were randomly assigned to either Quiet Mind Training or a control condition. Dart playing skills and alpha were assessed four times: at baseline, 20 session later, under stress conditions, and at study end.

In the penultimate study, this collection proposes that prefrontal neurofeedback training would be accompanied by changes in the relative power of EEG bands and ratios of individual bands with increased effectiveness at higher numbers of sessions. Outcome measures included EEG and behavioral ratings by parents/caregivers.

Mu rhythm and bimanual coordination was examined in 10 healthy boys, 10 boys with high-functioning in-active autism and 10 boys with high-functioning active autism. Results indicated that high-functioning in-active autistic boys and high-functioning active autistic boys have a higher mean of relative phase error.

Chapter 1 - This chapter presents a number of possible applications of neurofeedback in offender treatment. A global description of the method is presented, followed by a brief overview of the empirical evidence of its efficacy in specific treatment areas that are relevant for offender treatment. Neurofeedback can be applied as an additive treatment modality in various areas of offender treatment including domestic violence, various other forms of violent and anti-social behavior, certain forms of sexually abusive behavior, and criminal behavior of an obsessive–compulsive nature.

Chapter 2 - In order to accomplish a targeted impact of neurofeedback on specific cortical functions 'EEG-based local brain activity neurofeedback training' (EEG-LBA-NF) was developed by Bauer et al., (2011). With this approach an implemented algorithm automatically identifies and localizes EEG-sources in successive sLORETA solutions. Based on this information the feedback is exclusively controlled by EEG-generating sources within a selected cortical region of training (ROT): Positive feedback is given if a source is located in the ROT and suspended if no source is detectable in the selected area. In this way the influence of sources in the vicinity of the ROT is excluded. In order to individually and precisely locate and define the ROT the use of evoked potentials (EPs) of known local origin is described and recommended. In addition to an evaluation via behavioral effects, this approach also enables the determination of the specificity of individual neurofeedback-applications on a neurophysiological level. First applications in both the time- and the frequency-domain yielded promising results: Subjects were able to significantly increase the feedback rate whereas controls receiving sham feedback were not.

Chapter 3 - Spinal cord injuries (SCIs) demand particular attention; people with SCI report reduced quality of life and impairments in everyday life. The authors tested whether and if so to what extent neurofeedback or a physical training could, compared to a control condition, improve reaction time and balance as proxies for fine motor control in a sample of Iranian veterans with SCI. A total of 30 Iranian veterans with SCI were randomly assigned to the following study conditions: neurofeedback, physical training, or a control condition (conventional therapy). Both at the beginning and four weeks later, reaction times and balance were objectively measured. Compared to the control condition and over time, reaction times improved in the neurofeedback condition, while balance improved in the physical training condition. Compared to a conventional treatment condition, neurofeedback and physical training improved skills in specific areas of motor control. Thus, it appears that both neurofeedback and physical training should be introduced as routine interventions for patients with SCIs.

Chapter 4 - The use of neurofeedback is growing rapidly in sport performance enhancement. The aim of this study was to investigate the effect of neurofeedback training on motor performance and conscious motor processing of skilled dart players. The participants were 20 male skilled dart players. The research was conducted in five phases, include: Pre-test, training neurofeedback, posttest 1, under pressure test and posttest 2. Training neurofeedback was consisted of prevent training to the Alpha band frequency (8 to 12 Hz) in F4. To data analyze descriptive statistics and Mixed ANOVA was used. Results indicate the amount of conscious motor processing for neurofeedback training group decreased at post-test 1($p = 0.001$) and, under pressure test. However, this reduction was not observed in the control group. The dart throw points for neurofeedback training group and control group in the post-test 1 compare to per-test were enhanced but only neurofeedback group($p = 0.001$) be able preserve this increase in the under pressure test. This study indicates, there are influences among neurofeedback training, conscious motor processing and athletic performance. In other words, the neurofeedback training by reducing the conscious motor processing leads to the desired motor performance and creates automatic sense in the athlete

Chapter 5 - The use of neurofeedback is growing rapidly in sport psychology and sport performance. In the present study, the authors aimed to investigate the effect of neurofeedback training on self-talk and motor performance of elite volleyball players. The participants consisted of 15 male elite volleyball players. The study was performed in three stages: pre-test, neurofeedback training, and post-test. Neurofeedback training consisted of 1) sensorimotor rhythm enhancement and 2) prevention training to the frequency of 12Hz at T3. Both at the beginning and at the end of the study, self-talk and service scores were measured. Data were analyzed with paired t-test as well as descriptive statistics. The data analysis indicated that self-talk decreased in the group of elite players at the post-test. In addition, the service scores showed higher improvement for the group of elite players at the post test. The results of the present study indicate that neurofeedback training, inner self-talk (analysis of skill), and athletic performance are inter-related.

Chapter 6 - The aim of this chapter was to investigate the effect of Neurofeedback Training (NFT) on alpha power and performance of dart throw. A total of 20 elite dart players were randomly assigned either to the NFT, and a control condition. NFT consisted of training to achieve alpha-wave inhibition in F4, while participants in the control condition practiced dart playing with unrelated NFT. Dart playing skills and alpha were assessed four times: at baseline, 4 session later, under stress conditions, and at study end. Over time, alpha power and radial errors reduced, but more so in the NFT condition than in the control condition. Furthermore, performance in the NFT conditions also remained stable under stress. The results indicate that among elite dart players and compared to a control condition, NFT provide significant improvements in implicit motor skills. Importantly, dart performance under NFT conditions also remained stable under stress.

Chapter 7 - Neurofeedback training is a treatment modality of potential use for improving self-regulation skills in autism spectrum disorder (ASD). Multiple studies using neurofeedback to target symptoms of ASD have been made. These studies differ among themselves in the type of training (e.g., theta-to-beta ratio, coherence, etc.), topography (Cz or Pz), guidance by quantitative EEG (qEEG), and number of sessions (e.g., 20 vs. 30, etc.). In the authors' study, they proposed that prefrontal neurofeedback training would be accompanied by changes in relative power of EEG bands (e.g., 40 Hz-centered gamma band) and ratios of individual bands (e.g., theta-to-beta ratio); with increased effectiveness at higher number of sessions (e.g., 12 vs. 18 vs. 24 sessions). Outcome measures included EEG and behavioral ratings by parents/caregivers. In the first pilot study on 8 children with ASD (~17.4 yrs.) the authors used a 12 session-long course of neurofeedback from the AFz site, while on the second study of 18 children (~13.2 yrs.) the authors administered 18 sessions of prefrontal neurofeedback training. In the third pilot study, presently underway, the authors administered 24 sessions of neurofeedback. The protocol used training for wide band EEG amplitude suppression ("InhibitAll") with simultaneous upregulation of the index of 40 Hz-centered gamma activity. QEEG analysis at the training site was completed for each session of neurofeedback in order to determine the relative power of the individual bands (theta, low and high beta, and gamma) and their ratios (e.g., theta-to-low beta) within and between sessions. In all three studies the authors analyzed Aberrant Behavior Checklist (ABC) ratings by caregivers (pre- and post-treatment). The pilot study that used 12 sessions showed only a trend of progress across the sessions even though changes of individual EEG bands and their ratios during individual sessions were significant. The 18 session-long course showed more significant improvements both in behavioral and prefrontal qEEG measures. The authors found a significant reduction in Lethargy/Social Withdrawal subscale of the ABC and decrease in Hyperactivity scores. In the 24 session-long study children with ASD (N = 6) were only partially analyzed as the study is still in progress and targets recruitment of at least 12 subjects. The authors' experiments showed advantages of 18 sessions-long weekly prefrontal neurofeedback course over the 12 session-long course. Children with ASD in a more extended neurofeedback course currently underway showed even more promising improvements in targeted neurofeedback measures and in behavioral symptoms of aberrant behavior such as irritability, lethargy/social withdrawal and hyperactivity. Future research is needed to assess qEEG changes at other topographies using brain mapping, more prolonged courses, and using other outcome measures including behavioral evaluations to judge the clinical utility of prefrontal neurofeedback in children with ASD. The current series support a need to address various factors affecting outcome of neurofeedback-based intervention, specifically the question of length of treatment.

Chapter 8 - Children with autism spectrum disorder have been sought to face the lack of motor control in their physical activities, however, some scientists stated that the reason for this weakness is dysfunction in the mirror neuron. In this causal-comparative study, the mu rhythm and bimanual coordination was examined in 10 healthy, 10 high-functioning autism (HFA) in-active and 10 high- functioning autism (HFA) active boys. Participants performed bimanual in-phase and anti-phase movements with their wrists at two conditions including: 1) observation, and 2) execution, while EEG was recorded. Two-way mixed ANOVA was used to analyze differences between both outcome measures of HFA in-active vs. HFA active. Results indicated that HFA in-active and HFA active boys have higher mean of relative phase error ($P \leq 0.01$), moreover, have lower mean in mu suppression in both condition; observation ($P = 0.001$) and execution ($P = 0.001$). Results showed that a significant effect of condition for all groups. Findings confirm that HFA active boys performed bimanual coordination task more accurately. The authors have seen that when HFA boys perform bimanual coordination task, the mirror neuron activity has increased. These findings suggest that the special attention should be paid to motor activities in the treatment and the healing of HFA children.

In: Neurofeedback
Editor: Michael C. Hellinger

ISBN: 978-1-53615-167-1
© 2019 Nova Science Publishers, Inc.

Chapter 1

NEUROFEEDBACK AND OFFENDER TREATMENT

*Ron van Outsem**

Inforsa-Arkin, Amsterdam, the Netherlands

ABSTRACT

This chapter presents a number of possible applications of neurofeedback in offender treatment. A global description of the method is presented, followed by a brief overview of the empirical evidence of its efficacy in specific treatment areas that are relevant for offender treatment.

Neurofeedback can be applied as an additive treatment modality in various areas of offender treatment including domestic violence, various other forms of violent and anti-social behavior, certain forms of sexually abusive behavior, and criminal behavior of an obsessive–compulsive nature.

---

* Corresponding Author Email: ronvanoutsem@casema.nl.

WHAT IS NEUROFEEDBACK?

Neurofeedback is a type of biofeedback that uses electro-encephalography (EEG) to provide a signal that can be used by a person to receive feedback about his or her present cortical brain activity. It is also called neurotherapy, neurobiofeedback, or EEG biofeedback. The method makes use of real-time displays of EEG to illustrate cortical brain activity with the goal of controlling this activity, and thus reducing symptoms and/or enhancing mental capabilities. Sensors are placed on the scalp to measure activity. The measurements are displayed using video and/or sound. The process of neurofeedback is usually understood as being based on a form of operant and/or classical conditioning. When cortical brain activity changes in the direction desired by the therapist directing the treatment, a 'reward' feedback is given to the patient. When the change is in the opposite direction from what was intended, then either different feedback is given or the provision of otherwise attained 'reward' feedback is inhibited. Rewards, or reinforcements, can be as simple as a change in pitch of a tone or as complex as a certain type of movement of a character in a video game. EEG pattern targets are based on extrapolations from research describing normal and abnormal EEG patterns. Different structures within the cerebral cortex play crucial roles in the origin and/or manifestation of different kinds of behavior and of emotional responses (Demos, 2005; Evans & Arbarbanel, 1999). Various forms of psychopathology are closely associated with specific dysfunctions in these cortical structures (Demos, 2005; Evans & Arbarbanel, 1999). Neurofeedback aims at restoring the activity of these structures to the level and pattern that is present in the corresponding cortical structures of healthy individuals by way of the conditioning process described earlier. The beneficial effects of neurofeedback on behavior and emotion are understood to be a consequence of the fact that the patient's cerebral cortex is trained to function in ways that approximate those of symptom-free individuals.

Several types of neurofeedback, so-called training protocols, exist. Each training protocol has its own specific purpose, technique, and effect. Different protocols are used for the treatment of different conditions, or for the enhancement of different specific brain functions. Some protocols are aimed at the regulation of the activity of a specific region of the cerebral cortex, other protocols target multiple cortical regions simultaneously. There are protocols that focus on the regulation of a single type of brain rhythm (i.e., a brain rhythm that falls within a certain frequency range), while other protocols work with brain rhythms of multiple frequencies. While some protocols aim at stimulating certain activities of the brain, others aim at synchronizing these activities. Probably the most well-known neurofeedback protocol is the so-called Alpha training (or Deep State training) protocol. This protocol aims at attaining a state of profound relaxation by stimulating a specific type of (low frequency) brain activity that reads on the electroencephalogram as 'alpha waves' (7.5 - 12.5 Hz waves). Demos (2005) provides an extensive overview of all of these protocols, their techniques, and their effects.

Neurofeedback is mostly a non-verbal method, making it adequate for patients who do not express themselves easily verbally or who do not master the country's language sufficiently. The latter is an important advantage in multi-cultural societies since it makes the method suitable for patients of different cultures and languages (Kelley, 1997; Othmer, Othmer, & Kaiser, 1999).

Neurofeedback is still a rarely used treatment method in offender treatment and offender rehabilitation programs all over the world. The method is all but ignored despite of its reported success rates (Kwan, 2002; Quinn, Bodenhamer-Davis, & Koch, 2004). An important reason for this could be that there is a widespread belief that neurofeedback is not an evidence based treatment method. Therefore, many practitioners are reluctant to adopt it and many insurance companies and mental health care subsidizers are equally reluctant to finance it. The sometimes fanatical and uncritical manner, in which some publicists have presented neurofeedback to their audiences and readerships, often referring to research of insufficient scientific rigor, may also have contributed considerably to the skepsis concerning this method. Another reason why neurofeedback is ignored in the field of offender treatment could be that most psychologists, psychiatrists and other mental health care workers are trained to perceive anti-social and criminal behavior mostly as a result of a problematic development and/or traumatic experiences. They usually have learned that the most effective way to treat these phenomena is to influence their patient's perceptions, thought patterns, and emotional reactions with the use of spoken (and written) word, role play, and medication. Neurofeedback's basic approach, i.e., healthier thinking, feeling and behaving by way of stimulating the brain to function in a healthier manner, is usually quite alien to them. The often perceived incompatibility of neurofeedback's basic approach and the basic approaches of traditional forms of psychotherapy may also account for some of the reluctance in the field to adopt this treatment method.

NEUROFEEDBACK IN THE LITERATURE THAT IS RELEVANT TO OFFENDER TREATMENT

In a review of 31 research publications concerning the efficacy of neurofeedback in areas that are relevant to offender treatment (Van Outsem, 2011), beneficial effects of neurofeedback treatment were reported in all publications. In none of the studies that were reviewed, grounds were found to designate neurofeedback as a totally ineffective treatment method. Negative effects, or side effects, were found to be absent in 25 of the 31 publications. In the remaining six publications, the presence or absence of negative effects was not discussed.

The attrition rates of neurofeedback treatment that were reported in the reviewed publications were considerably lower than what is usual in most of the current forms of psychotherapy. While attrition rates of 30 – 50% are very common among current forms of offender treatment (Van Wijk et al., 2007; Wilson & Cumming, 2009), the average attrition rate for neurofeedback treatment is found to be only around 15%.

In the reviewed publications in which neurofeedback was compared to other treatment methods, the reported success rates of neurofeedback exceeded those of the other methods, including cognitive behavioral therapy and medication (Gruzelier & Egner, 2005; Hammond, 2003; McKnight & Fehmi, 2001; Vernon et al., 2004). This was also the case when the effects were evaluated again after a follow-up period of 1–5 years (Butnik, 2005; Evans & Arbarbanel, 1999; Gruzelier & Egner, 2005; McKnight & Fehmi, 2001; Scott et al., 2002; Quinn et al., 2004; Vernon et al., 2004). However, because of the relatively small number of comparative studies that are conducted to date, one should be careful to draw definitive conclusions as to the efficacy of neurofeedback in comparison to other treatment methods in a considerable number of areas.

When investigating the efficacy of any method of treatment, it is necessary to assess the role of factors that are not specific to the treatment method itself, but which nonetheless may influence the measurements of its effects. Three of such factors, which are very important are the placebo effect, the patient–therapist relationship, and the therapist's personal qualities. In the conducted review, two studies on the efficacy of neurofeedback were found which referred specifically to the role of these non-specific factors. Engelbrecht et al. (2010) concluded from their placebo controlled study that changes in EEG patterns after treatment were to be attributed to the neurofeedback program itself, and not to any extent to the placebo effect. In this study, no post treatment changes in EEG patterns were found in the placebo group. Conversely, the intended changes were found in the treatment group. The subjects in the placebo group had completed a sham neurofeedback program. According to the authors, all subjects were convinced that they had followed the real neurofeedback treatment. McKnight and Fehmi (2001) found in their evaluative study that the health benefits of neurofeedback that were reported by their subjects were independent of the skill or experience of the therapist who treated them. Also, no correlation was found between the treatment outcome and the reported quality of the relationship between therapist and patient. These findings are consistent with the premise that the effects of neurofeedback are not the result of non-specific factors. They rather constitute support for the efficacy of the treatment program itself.

To date, there is insufficient evidence to be found in the literature that neurofeedback could reduce aggressive and/or anti-social behavior in patients suffering from personality disorders. Personality disorders are regularly diagnosed among forensic patients (Nestor, 2002). The possibility exists, however, that this treatment method could alleviate some of the symptoms that are associated with the various types of personality disorders. Further research in this area is needed to determine whether, and if so to what extent, neurofeedback can be of value in the treatment of forensic patients suffering from personality disorders. Valid research on the effects of neurofeedback in patients suffering from psychotic disorders like schizophrenia is also still scarce. So far, it cannot be determined whether neurofeedback could be of any use in the treatment of psychotic forensic patients.

In most of the reviewed publications, it is not in any way advocated that neurofeedback should replace traditional forms of psychotherapy altogether in the areas of treatment for which evidence of neurofeedback's efficacy exists. While neurofeedback may create an ability in the patient to achieve behavioral and emotional change by optimizing certain brain functions, other forms of psychotherapy, e.g., cognitive behavioral therapy, can provide guidance as to the directions in which this change could take place. For instance, partial or total recovery from (long-term) addiction and/or psychopathology often places the patient in a situation in which a new personal life-style has to be developed. The patient may change his/her choice of friends, change his/her way of relating to other people, take up a new career, etc. Counseling is generally considered as being very useful when a patient stands before the challenge of designing and adopting a new personal life-style. Therefore, neurofeedback and traditional forms of psychotherapy should be seen as complementary partners rather than as competitors.

SUDS AND ADHD

Substance Use Disorders (SUDs) and Attention Deficit/Hyperactivity Disorder (ADHD) are both important contributing factors in the development and exacerbation of many different kinds of antisocial and criminal behavior. They are also significant hampering factors in offender treatment, leading to a high rate of attrition, a low level of compliance to treatment, and a decreased ability in the patient to integrate new insights, new skills, and alternative behavior patterns ('t Hart- Kerkhoffs, 2010; Vermeiren, 2002; Wilson & Cumming, 2009). Treatment success in antisocial patients suffering from SUDs and/or ADHD is indeed a very rare phenomenon (Adshead & Brown, 2003; Van Outsem, 2009; Weijers, 2008; Wilson & Cumming, 2009). ADHD and SUDs are conditions that are often found among forensic patients, both juveniles and adults (Adshead & Brown, 2003; Van Wijk, 2005; Vermeiren, 2002; Welldon & Van Velsen, 1996; Wilson & Cumming, 2009).

Offender treatment as a whole faces many challenges. First of all, most treatment outcome studies in the forensic field reveal only limited sized effects, if any effects at all (Atkinson, 1999; Babcock & Steiner, 1999; Chambers et al., 2008; Craissati, et al., 2009; Gondolf, 1997; Gordon & Moriarty, 2003; Hanson et al., 2002; Hanson et al., 2003; Kohl & Macy, 2008; Lin et al., 2009; Loeber et al., 2001; Macy et al., 2010; Marshall et al., 1999; Peek & Nugter, 2009; Plichta & Falik, 2001; Seager et al., 2004; Van Wijk et al., 2007; Weijers, 2008). Consequently, the current forms of psychotherapy seem to be of only limited value in the efforts to prevent re-offense. Second, there is the problem of attrition and therapy compliance, not only in the patients suffering from SUDs and/or ADHD. In offender treatment, overall attrition rates tend to be very high and treatment compliance levels very low (Beech et al., 1998; Chambers et al., 2008; Lin et al., 2009; Loeber et al., 2001; Marshall et al., 1999; Miner, 2002; Peek & Nugter, 2009; Ryan & Lane, 1997; Seager et al., 2004; Van Outsem, 2009; Van Wijk et al., 2007; Weijers, 2008). In this respect, the problem of low compliance rates of medication intake, especially in patients with ADHD, should be noted. Third, many (forensic) patients have great difficulty in discussing their thoughts, feelings, and experiences adequately enough for psychotherapy to be fruitful. Among the main reasons for this are mistrust, shame, lack of introspective abilities, weakness of verbal expression, and cognitive disabilities (Van Outsem, 2009). Finally, especially in multicultural societies, there is the problem of language barriers. Insufficient mastering of the language in which the treatment is conducted can be a major problem in conducting the treatment successfully. It can be concluded that new approaches in offender treatment are needed to overcome these problems.

Recent advances in neuropsychology, however, offer new perspectives on the treatment of patients who frequently display antisocial and criminal behavior and who suffer from SUDs and/or ADHD. One of these recent advances are those in the field of neurofeedback.

EMPIRICAL SUPPORT FOR THE EFFICACY OF NEUROFEEDBACK IN ADHD AND SUDS

The two areas of treatment in which neurofeedback's efficacy is most empirically supported, and which are relevant for offender treatment, are ADHD and SUDs.

ADHD

In this area, the efficacy of neurofeedback is well established and documented (Arns et al., 2009; Butnik, 2005; Carmody et al., 2001; Fuchs et al., 2003; Gruzelier & Egner, 2005; Heinrich et al., 2004; Kaiser & Othmer, 2000; Linden et al., 1996; Lubar & Lubar, 1999; Masterpasqual & Healey, 2003; Monastra et al., 2002; Monastra et al., 2005; Nash, 2000; Patrick, 1996; Robbins, 2000; Rossiter & La Vaque, 1995; Schulenburg, 1999; Thompson & Thompson, 1998; Tinius & Tinius, 2000; Vernon et al., 2004). In these publications, a total of 1232 subjects were studied. Randomized controlled trials are the most prevalent in this area of treatment (five studies). Heterogeneity was not significant (I^2 = .22, p = .15). No significant publication bias was found (Egger's p = .9). Symptom reduction was found in patients of all age groups. Around 80% of patients show measurable improvements, which, in most studies, are corroborated by parents, teachers, and/or spouses. These improvements consist of increases in concentration and self-control and of the amelioration of social behavior in general. The social behavior of the treated patients tends to become more empathic, while impulsive and aggressive behavior toward others significantly decreases. The magnitude of the desired effects of neurofeedback in patients with ADHD is at least comparable to that of stimulant medication therapy, and is in many cases greater (Arns et al., 2009; Fuchs et al., 2003; Gruzelier & Egner, 2005; Heinrich et al., 2004; Kaiser & Othmer, 2000; Linden et al., 1996; Monastra et al., 2002, 2005; Rossiter & La Vaque, 1995). Arns et al. (2009) concluded from their meta-analytic study that neurofeedback can be considered efficacious and specific as a treatment for ADHD since both prospective controlled studies and studies employing a pre- and post-design found large effect sizes for neurofeedback on impulsivity and inattention, for both Hedges' $\hat{g}$ = .8, and medium effect sizes on hyperactivity, Hedges' $\hat{g}$ = .6. Most authors name as an important advantage of neurofeedback over stimulant medication treatment for ADHD that the desired effects remain for a prolonged period of time after treatment, and that these effects are often permanent (Arns et al., 2009; Fuchs et al., 2003; Gruzelier& Egner, 2005; Heinrich et al., 2004; Kaiser & Othmer, 2000; Linden et al., 1996; Monastra et al., 2002, 2005; Rossiter & La Vaque, 1995; Schulenburg, 1999; Thompson & Thompson, 1998; Vernon et al., 2004). Conversely, the effects of stimulant medication end when the intake of these substances ends. Moreover, the often present side effects of stimulant medication, which have a strong negative effect on compliance with this type of treatment, are totally absent when neurofeedback is applied (Fuchs et al., 2003; Gruzelier & Egner, 2005; Kaiser & Othmer, 2000; Monastra et al., 2002, 2005; Rossiter & La Vaque,

1995; Vernon et al., 2004). The temporary worsening of symptoms of ADHD when medication is not taken on time, the so-called rebound effect, is also not a problem when neurofeedback treatment is chosen (Fuchs et al., 2003; Gruzelier & Egner, 2005; Heinrich et al., 2004; Kaiser & Othmer, 2000; Rossiter & La Vaque, 1995). The advantages of neurofeedback over stimulant medication therapy in patients with ADHD are especially eminent in the light of the fact that in stimulant medication therapy compliance is usually very low and attrition very high (Fuchs et al., 2003; Gruzelier & Egner, 2005; Linden et al., 1996; Monastra et al., 2002, 2005; Rossiter & La Vaque, 1995).

SUDs

Considerable documentation on neurofeedback's effectiveness in the area of alcohol and drug dependency can be found in the literature (Burkett et al., 2005; Kelley, 1997; Peniston & Kulkoski, 1999; Scott et al., 2002; Scott et al., 2005; Quinn et al., 2004; Trudeau, 2000). In the studies of abstinence (0 – 4 uses after completion of treatment) versus relapse (more than four uses after treatment completion) during a follow-up period of 1 – 5 years, the computed effect sizes (odds ratio) ranged between 4.1 (crack cocaine, 1-year follow-up) and 6.7 (alcohol, 5 years follow-up). Effect sizes in studies on the self-reported number of uses during 1 – 5 years after treatment completion ranged between Hedges' $\hat{g} = .6$ (crack cocaine, 1-year follow-up) and .9 (alcohol, 5 years follow-up). According to four studies, the efficacy of neurofeedback exceeds that of current treatment methods in this area after a follow-up period of 1 – 5 years (Burkett et al., 2005; Callaway & Bodenhamer-Davis, E., 2008; Quinn et al., 2004; Trudeau, 2000). After completion of conventional forms of substance abuse treatment, 65 – 70% of patients take (any amount of) alcohol or drugs again within the first year (McKay et al., 1999). For neurofeedback treatment, this rate is 45–50% (Burkett et al., 2005; Quinn et al., 2004; Trudeau, 2000). Of the evaluative studies that were selected on neurofeedback as a treatment method for alcohol and drug dependency, three were randomized controlled studies. Significant heterogeneity (I^2 = .79, p = .002) was found. This was caused by the fact that patients with different types of addiction were studied. Relapse in crack cocaine addiction was considerably more prevalent than in addiction to alcohol or marijuana. No significant publication bias (Egger's p = .4) was found. A total of 511 subjects participated in these studies.

Two large studies in Texas (Callaway & Bodenhamer-Davis, 2008) showed quite remarkable results. One study was done within the state corrections system, the other with addicted homeless people (95% of whom were crack cocaine addicts). Three-year follow-up data was strongly indicative of success using the neurofeedback treatment. Sixty-nine patients completed treatment and have been followed for from six months to one and one-half years after treatment. Success was defined very stringently, through four criteria, all of which had to be met:

1. Not on drugs (verified though random urine analysis).
2. Not homeless.
3. Not unemployed (at work or in school).
4. Not arrested.

None of these patients were employed or had a home when they entered treatment, and all had lengthy police records. After one and one-half years 83% of patients were successful in meeting all four criteria.

POSSIBLE APPLICATIONS OF NEUROFEEDBACK IN OFFENDER TREATMENT

According to the literature, neurofeedback could play a role in the following areas of offender treatment:

Aggression, Anti-Social, and Criminal Behavior Related to Substance Abuse

Substance abuse, especially the abuse of alcohol, opiates, cocaine, and amphetamines, is a well-known cause, catalyst, and perpetuator of aggressive, anti-social, and criminal behavior such as theft, burglary, street-robbery, physical and sexual violence, drug trafficking, etc. (Glass, 1991; Martin & Johnson, 2005; Nestor, 2002; Wekerle & Wall, 2002). In most of these cases, solving the substance dependency problem is tantamount to solving the total behavior problem (Glass, 1991; Wekerle & Wall, 2002). Since neurofeedback has shown good results in helping patients to recover from their addiction and to stay abstinent, it should be seriously considered when substance abuse is a pivotal factor in the patient's problem behavior.

Domestic Violence

In the field of domestic violence, there are several processes in which neurofeedback could prove helpful. First, there is again the problem of substance abuse. The abuse of alcohol is by far the most powerful predictor of re-offense after treatment in domestic violence offenders (Lin et al., 2009). Second, much of the violent behavior within intimate relationships is caused by conditioned emotional responses to cues, which are interpreted as a confirmation of certain aversive cognitions (Dutton, 2006; Hamel & Nicholls, 2007; Hampton et al., 2006; Jackson, 2007; McCue, 2008; Van Outsem, 2001). The most common of these responses are pathological jealousy (a strong emotional response to a perceived confirmation of the thought that the subject's partner is being unfaithful), fear of abandonment (which occurs strongly when the subject perceives any cue as a sign that his/her partner is planning to leave him/her), and sense of disqualification (a strong response of anger and humiliation when the subject perceives any cue as a confirmation of his/her conviction that his/her partner does not take the subject seriously, does not care for the subject, or puts the subject's abilities into question). Neurofeedback could be used here as a tool to enhance the subject's flexibility of thinking and of emotional response as is described by McKnight and Fehmi (2001). As a result, the patient may become more able to challenge and modulate his/her own negative cognitions and to generate more constructive behavioral responses to perceived negative cues. Third, again as described by McKnight and Fehmi (2001), neurofeedback could be effective in relieving stress, which results from the unconscious effort to maintain habitual forms of focused attention. This translates into the stress which is experienced in daily life and which is usually accompanied by the phenomena of rumination and 'gripping' (i.e., hyperfocusing on stress-provoking cues). These phenomena often play an important role in fuelling domestic violence (Dutton, 2006; Hamel & Nicholls, 2007; Hampton et al., 2006; Jackson, 2007; McCue, 2008; Van Outsem, 2001). The enhancement of flexibility of thinking and of emotional response is also here a key process of recovery.

Neurofeedback may also be a valuable tool in the treatment of other forms of violent and anti-social behavior, i.e., that takes place outside intimate relationships, in which an important role is played by the phenomena that are mentioned above.

Aggression Problems and Delinquency Caused By, or Catalyzed by, Attention Deficit Hyperactivity Disorder (ADHD)

Aggression problems and criminal behavior are often a part of the total problem behavior that is displayed by patients suffering from ADHD ('t Hart-Kerkhoffs, 2010; Peniston et al., 1993; Vermeiren, 2002; Wilson & Cumming, 2009). The efficacy of neurofeedback in treating ADHD, as is reported in the literature, may offer possibilities for the reduction of the impulsive aggressive behavior that is often associated with this condition. This may especially be the case in patients who do not react satisfactorily to medication or who fail to comply with the medication regime.

Aggression Problems and Delinquency Caused By, or Catalyzed by, Autism Spectrum Disorder (ASD) and Post Traumatic Stress Disorder (PTSD)

These disorders are also sometimes accompanied by aggressive outbursts and delinquent behavior ('t Hart-Kerkhoffs, 2010; Vermeiren, 2002; Wilson & Cumming, 2009). The efficacy of neurofeedback in treating these specific conditions is less empirically supported than that in treating ADHD and SUDs, although some evidence does exist (Kouijzer et al., 2008; Martin & Johnson, 2005; Peniston et al., 1991, 1993; Peterson, 2000; Smith & Sams, 2005; Van Outsem, 2011).

Prevention of Delinquent Behavior

Neurofeedback could also play a role in the *prevention* of criminal behavior. The early treatment of conditions such as ADHD, Post Traumatic Stress Disorder (PTSD), and SUDs could probably reduce the probability of development of criminal behavior in (young) patients who are treated successfully. Also, the treatment of learning difficulties with the use of neurofeedback may, at least to some extent, prevent drop-out from school. This may also have a preventive effect on delinquency. According to a growing body of research, neurofeedback offers good results in the treatment of various types of learning disabilities (Fenger, 1998; Fernández et al., 2003; Hammond, 2007; Tansey, 1991; Thompson & Thompson, 1998)

THE PRACTICE OF NEUROFEEDBACK

First of all, neurofeedback, unfortunately, is not for everybody. Several exclusion criteria for the method are found in the literature. These exclusion criteria are related to the occurrence of adverse effects and/or symptom exacerbation in the patient when applying the treatment. General consensus exists on the following exclusion criteria:

- The diagnosis of schizophrenia and/or psychotic episodes in the patient's history.
- The diagnosis of borderline personality disorder.
- The diagnosis of bipolar disorder.
- The current daily use of significant quantities of alcohol and/or the frequent use of drugs. Patients suffering from SUDs need to be abstinent for at least one month before neurofeedback treatment can be administered. The detoxification phase of SUDs treatment needs to be completed before starting neurofeedback.

A neurofeedback treatment is usually completed after 30–60 sessions, depending on the severity of the symptoms that are treated and on the pace with which the patient's brain reacts to the treatment. Usually the treatment is discontinued if no change in the EEG readings is found after 10–15 sessions. The reason for this is that, in most cases, no further effects are to be expected if changes remain absent after 10 – 15 sessions (Demos, 2005). Neurofeedback can be incorporated in both inpatient and outpatient treatment programs. The frequency of the sessions can vary between once a week and four sessions a day. A typical neurofeedback session takes about thirty minutes to complete.

The application of neurofeedback protocols is relatively easy to be trained in for licensed psychotherapists and psychiatrists. Neurofeedback courses are available in a growing number of countries. There are also good quality neurofeedback courses to be found online.

High-quality neurofeedback equipment is easy to acquire and is quite affordable for most practitioners. A complete high-quality neurofeedback system should not cost more than three thousand U.S. dollars. Additional requirements include:

- A laptop computer.
- A comfortable chair for the patient to sit in.

- A second computer screen.
- A quiet room.

A typical neurofeedback session consists of the following elements:

1. The patient is welcomed.
2. The patient is briefly asked about his/her current emotional and physical state, about any recent consumption of alcohol or drugs, about any important recent events that may affect neurofeedback training, and about any positive or adverse effects the patient experiences during the neurofeedback treatment. The session will be cancelled if the patient is under the influence of alcohol and/or drugs, or if the patient is hung-over after consuming alcohol or drugs the previous day. The session will also be cancelled if the patient reports adverse effects of the treatment. In this case, it will be discussed with the patient whether the treatment will be continued using another protocol or whether the treatment will be discontinued altogether.
3. The patient is seated in the training chair and the electrodes are attached to the patient's head. This is done using a sticky paste that is a good conductor of electricity. Before attaching the electrodes, the specific locations on the scalp where the electrodes are placed are scrubbed gently using a special scrubbing gel. This is called a skin preparation gel.
4. The neurofeedback training is conducted, usually for a period of twenty minutes. With many patients, it is advisable to take a one-minute break halfway the training session. With some patients, a one-minute brake once every five minutes is necessary.
5. When the training is finished, the electrodes are removed from the patient's head and the remaining conductive paste is wiped off the patient's scalp and hair.
6. The course of the training is discussed with the patient. The patient is asked about his/her emotional state and the session is concluded.

It is inadvisable to combine psychotherapy and neurofeedback in one session. Although neurofeedback and psychotherapy are a complementary combination, conducting both psychotherapy and neurofeedback within the same session is often experienced as too fatiguing by many patients. Therefore, neurofeedback and psychotherapy should be conducted in separate sessions.

NEUROFEEDBACK IN ADHD

The neurofeedback protocols that are used in treating ADHD are all so-called qEEG-guided, or qEEG-informed, protocols. These are protocols that are based on the result of the patient's qEEG.

The qEEG (quantitative electroencephalogram) is also known in popular terms as a "brain map". An electroencephalogram is a report on electrical activity within the brain that provides detailed information about brain function. The report is produced by a biomedical device called an electroencephalograph. A quantitative EEG differs from a traditional EEG in that it performs an extensive set of computerized statistical analyses on the collected raw EEG data. The EEG patterns from an individual's brain are compared with a normative database containing data from a large number of other individual EEGs. The EEG data within this database are collected from a group of carefully-selected, symptom free, healthy people of different age groups. The individual's EEG is always compared to the EEG data in the normative database of other individuals in a similar age group. This statistically analyzed EEG, the qEEG, provides the clinician with a great deal more specific information about brain function than a traditional EEG.

Important kinds of information quantified by the qEEG include:

- A measure of the amount of electrical activity (in a range of different frequency bands) at many standardized scalp locations. This information is called a "power analysis".

- A measure of the nature of the connections, or communication pathways, between different locations on the brain's cortex. This information is called a "coherence analysis".

More in-depth information about the qEEG is found in the introductory book by John Demos (2005). Interpreting a qEEG is a complex matter with a steep learning curve. However, it is also possible for the clinician to only collect the raw EEG data and to have them analyzed by specialized professionals. These professionals will usually also provide the neurofeedback treatment protocol to be used based on the qEEG report.

In treating ADHD with neurofeedback, qEEG-guided protocols are preferred to standard protocols. The reason for this is that different variants of dysfunctional EEG patterns exist within the group of patients suffering from ADHD. The two most common EEG patterns found in ADHD patients are:

- Frontal slowing: This is an excess of slow synchronized activity in the range of 1 to 12 Hz located in the frontal areas of the cerebral cortex. Around 70% of patients suffering from ADHD show this EEG pattern (Thompson & Thompson, 2003).
- Diffuse Beta: This is an excess of fast desynchronized activity (usually above 20 Hz) that is found over the entire cerebral cortex. This pattern is found in about 20% of all ADHD patients (Thompson & Thompson 2003).

The remaining 10% of ADHD patients show various kinds of atypical EEG patterns.

In the case of frontal slowing, most qEEG-guided neurofeedback protocols that are used target frontal, prefrontal and central cortical areas and are designed to reduce slow frontal activity and to enhance faster desynchronized frontal activity. In the case of the diffuse Beta variant, the protocols that are most frequently used target central and parietal cortical areas. These protocols are designed to eliminate the excessive fast and desynchronized cortical activity. The general idea is to customize the neurofeedback protocol so that it stimulates every individual patient's brain to counteract its own specific dysfunctional cortical activity pattern.

NEUROFEEDBACK IN SUDS

Patients suffering from SUDs are eligible for neurofeedback treatment when they are abstinent for at least one month. The detoxification phase of SUDs treatment needs to be fully completed before starting neurofeedback.

The best empirically supported neurofeedback protocol is the Peniston protocol with the Scott and Kaiser modifications (Bodenhamer-Davis & Callaway, 2004; Callaway & Bodenhamer-Davis, 2008; Scott et al., 2005; Sokhadze et al., 2008). Several slightly different versions of this protocol exist.

A Neurofeedback Protocol for the Treatment of SUDs

This protocol is based on the Peniston protocol with the Scott and Kaiser modifications. It is one of the many variants of it that exist.

After the completion of detoxification (i.e., at least a month after attaining stable and complete abstinence), and when all diagnostic conclusions are reached, the patients have several (at least two) sessions with the neurofeedback therapist in which the following subjects are discussed:

- General information about neurofeedback.
- What the patient can and cannot expect from neurofeedback treatment.
- The necessity of psychotherapy next to neurofeedback (neurofeedback *is not an alternative for* psychotherapy. Neurofeedback and psychotherapy are complementary treatment modalities).

- What is expected from the patient (total abstinence during treatment, attending all sessions, reporting adverse effects, reporting relapse, etc.).
- What the neurofeedback training sessions are like.
- The expected number of sessions, the planning of the sessions during the week, and the time-span of the complete neurofeedback treatment.
- Any questions the patient may have.
- How to use the symptom and craving self report diary.

During neurofeedback treatment, the patients keep a self report diary in which subjective progress in terms of symptoms and craving is monitored. It is generally considered useful to employ rating scales to quantify subjective symptoms and craving.

Before starting the neurofeedback treatment, the therapist and the patient write three to five so-called vignettes. These vignettes are short patient-personalized stories about successfully rejecting alcohol and/or drugs.

When all preparations are completed, the neurofeedback sessions will start. The applied treatment protocol is a standard neurofeedback protocol, so no qEEG is required. The protocol comprises two phases:

Phase 1

In phase one, fifteen to twenty sessions of Sensory Motor Rhythm (SMR) and Theta training will take place. In these sessions, the augmentation of the production of SMR (12-15 Hz activity) on the Cz location (one channel) or C3 and C4 locations (two channels) is rewarded. Simultaneously, the decrease of the production of Theta (4-8 Hz activity) at Cz or C3 and C4 is also rewarded. The designated scalp locations are in accordance with the International 10-20 system of electrode application.

Phase 2

In phase two, twenty sessions of Alpha-Theta training is administered. The patient is rewarded when the power of Theta (4-8 Hz activity) exceeds that of Alpha (8-12 Hz activity) at the scalp locations Pz (one channel) or P3 and P4 (two channels). Immediately before starting the training, one of the vignettes is read to the patient by the therapist. The patient is instructed to imagine the vignette as vividly as possible.

VIGNETTES

Vignettes are written according to the following criteria:

- Vignettes are short. They take no longer than one minute to be read.
- The vignettes describe situations that are common risk situations in the patient's daily life.
- The vignettes are written in the patient's own words.
- The type of alcoholic beverage the patient typically drinks and/or drug the patient is addicted to is explicited. These substances are referred to using the names the patient uses for them.
- The vignettes have the following basic structure: 1: the description of the risk situation, 2: the description of the experience of temptation and craving, 3: the overcoming of the temptation and the craving, and 4: the experience of positive emotions as a result of overcoming the situation.

SOME EXAMPLES OF VIGNETTES

Vignette "Yesterday's Friends"

Imagine yourself walking down a street in your neighborhood. Suddenly you see a couple of old friends you used to drink/do drugs with (specify the drug the patient is addicted to). You have a very nice talk with them, reviving old memories of the good old "wild" times.

One of your old friends then says he knows about a great party taking place tonight. It's just the kind of party you used to go to and enjoy together with your old friends. The idea is born to meet up at this old friend's house, have a drink and a _____ (specify drug) first, and then go to the party. Everybody is very enthusiastic about the idea. You know you do have the money to go to this party. You really feel the temptation to go.

Then suddenly you start getting second thoughts about going to the party. Of course you like seeing your old friends again. Of course you would like to party again. Of course you would like to have a drink/use some _____ (specify drug) again. You feel your heart is racing. You feel the craving again!

But then you start thinking about your addiction. You realize that going to this party is a very risky thing. This party could mean total relapse. You start thinking about your addiction and about all the problems it has brought you in your life. You start thinking about how unhappy your addiction has made you feel.

Then you hear the voice of your conscience. It sounds a lot louder and convincing than usual. It's a warm and friendly voice that tells you to imagine how happy you would be without the alcohol/_____ (specify drug). You start thinking about all the things you could do without the addiction holding you back. You feel that your craving for the alcohol/_____ (specify drug) is getting less and less, until it goes away completely. You start feeling calm, happy and confident!

You tell your old friends that you are not going to the party this evening and you explain to them why. You are not affected in any way by their protests and objections. You don't mind being called a party crasher or a wet blanket. You don't care if they say you will miss out on an awesome night. You don't care that they say that they won't have so much fun without you....you don't feel guilty about it.

You walk away feeling happy and proud of yourself. You feel like a winner!

Vignette "The Liquor Store"

On a Saturday afternoon you walk past a liquor store. You can't help noticing an advertisement-board in the window. Your favorite drink is on sale! This week only, you can buy two whole bottles of _____ _____ (specify product, brand and type/variant) for the price of one. You look at the big full color picture of the _____ (specify). It looks tempting and delicious! You really feel like entering the liquor store and buy your _____ (specify).

Your heart is racing. You can taste the _____ (specify) in your mouth. You really feel the craving for the _____ (specify).

Then you hear the voice of your conscience. It sounds a lot louder and convincing than usual. It's a warm and friendly voice that tells you to imagine how happy you would be without the alcohol/_____ (specify). You start thinking about all the things you could do without the addiction holding you back. You feel that your craving for the alcohol/_____ (specify) is getting less and less, until it goes away completely. You start feeling calm, happy and confident!

You decide not to go in and by any alcohol. You feel strong and confident. You think of all the things you can do without your addiction to alcohol.

You walk away feeling happy and proud of yourself. You feel like a winner!

Vignette "In the Bar"

You know it probably wasn't a very good idea, but you agreed to go to a bar with some friends. You may even have thought that this was a good opportunity to prove to yourself and to your friends that you could stay off the booze even in very tempting situations.

You enter the bar and you see a lot of old friends you used to have good times with. You engage in very nice conversations with them and you drink only Coca Cola or mineral water. You feel proud that you haven't given in to the temptation to drink alcohol.

It's getting later and later, and you are getting a bit tired. Everybody else is clearly having a lot of fun. Everybody is drinking alcohol, some people obviously quite a lot! You are starting to feel a little lonesome. You are considering going home, but you feel bad to go home before your friends do. They are having a lot of fun. You feel you **don't** fit in the party.

Before you know it, you begin saying things to yourself like "Well, one drink won't hurt". Or "I have been sober for months, having one drink doesn't mean I'll relapse".

Then you hear the voice of your conscience. It sounds a lot louder and convincing than usual. It's a warm and friendly voice that tells you to imagine how happy you would be without the alcohol. You start thinking about all the things you could do without the addiction holding you back. You feel that your craving for the alcohol is getting less and less, until it goes away completely. You start feeling calm, happy and confident!

You decide to call it a night and to go home. You feel strong and confident. You think of all the things you can do without your addiction to alcohol.

You walk away feeling happy and proud of yourself. You feel like a winner!

Vignette "Home Alone"

You are home alone. You feel very bored, you have nothing to do. Actually, you don't really feel like doing anything. There is no one you can call or meet up with. You watch some television and make some coffee. You walk a bit about the house, you feel very, very bored. This feeling of emptiness is really getting to you.

Your old medicine for these kind of situations was having a _____ (specify drink or drug). This really made you feel better, more relaxed, more energetic, more self-confident. That empty feeling used to go away after having a _____ (specify). Life seemed a lot more fun when having a _____ (specify) was still OK.

You can't get your mind off having a _____ (specify). Your heart starts racing. You really feel the craving for a _____ (specify).

Then you hear the voice of your conscience. It sounds a lot louder and convincing than usual. It's a warm and friendly voice that tells you to imagine how happy you would be without the _____ (specify). You start thinking about all the things you could do without the addiction holding you back. You feel that your craving for the _____ (specify) is getting less and less, until it goes away completely. You start feeling calm, happy and confident!

You decide not to have a _____ (specify) but to call an old friend or family member instead. You feel strong and confident. You think of all the things you can do without your addiction to _____ (specify).

You feel happy and proud of yourself. You feel like a winner!

Vignette "Quarrel with the Wife/Husband"

Again you had a fight with your wife/husband/boyfriend/girlfriend. The fights are always about the same problems that just seem unsolvable. These problems, and fights, just keep coming back.

You are very angry with your wife/husband/boyfriend/girlfriend. You feel that he/she isn't doing enough to make your relationship better. Sometimes you get the impression that he/she doesn't really care anymore. Maybe his/her love for you is ebbing away, maybe he/she doesn't love you anymore. You're feeling angry and sad at the same time. Sometimes you even feel desperate and powerless. You just don't know what to do anymore.

You feel consumed by all these bad feelings and want to get away from it all. You really want to have a _____ (specify drink or drug). After all, who cares anymore? Having a _____ (specify) now seems the only way out of all this. You may even feel you have the right to have a

_____ (specify) because of the way your wife/husband/ boyfriend/girlfriend makes you feel.

Then you hear the voice of your conscience. It sounds a lot louder and convincing than usual. It's a warm and friendly voice that tells you to imagine how happy you would be without the _____ (specify). You start thinking about all the things you could do without the addiction holding you back. You feel that your craving for the _____ (specify) is getting less and less, until it goes away completely. You start feeling calm, happy and confident!

You decide not to have a _____ (specify) but to call a good friend or a family member to talk about the problems in your relationship. Maybe you'll get some good advice about what to do. You feel strong and confident. You think of all the things you can do without your addiction to _____ (specify). You feel happy and proud of yourself. You feel like a winner!

Completion of the Neurofeedback Treatment

When phases one and two are completed, the neurofeedback treatment is completed. The treatment is evaluated as to its results and further treatment is discussed with the patient.

CONCLUSION

Neurofeedback is still a relatively young method of treatment. Fortunately, scientific research and innovational activities in this field have gained considerable momentum during de past two decades. It is therefore to be expected that the efficacy and applicability of neurofeedback will continue to grow and that the method will eventually earn recognition as a valuable form of offender treatment.

REFERENCES

Adshead, G. & Brown, C. (2003). *Ethical issues in forensic mental health research*. London: Jessica Kingsley.

Arns, M., De Ridder, S., Strehl, U., Breteler, M. & Coenen, T. (2009). Efficacy of neurofeedback treatment in ADHD: The effects on inattention, impulsivity and hyperactivity. A meta-analysis. *EEG and Clinical Neuroscience*, *40*, 180–189.

Atkinson, B. (1999). The emotional imperative psychotherapists cannot afford to ignore. *Family Therapy Networker*, *23*, 22–33.

Babcock, J. C. & Steiner, R. (1999). The relationship between treatment, incarceration, and recidivism of battering: A program evaluation of Seattle's coordinated community response to domestic violence. *Journal of Family Psychology*, *13*(1), 23–34.

Beech, A., Fisher, D. & Beckett, R. (1998). *STEP-3: An evaluation of the prison sex offender treatment programme*. Oxford: Oxford Regional Forensic Service.

Bodenhamer-Davis, E. & Callaway, T. (2004). Extended follow-up of Peniston protocol results with chemical dependency. *Journal of Neurotherapy*, *8* (2), 135.

Burkett, V. S., Cummins, J. M., Dickson, R. M. & Skolnick, M. (2005). An open clinical trial utilizing real-time EEG operant conditioning as an adjunctive therapy in the treatment of crack cocaine dependence. *Journal of Neurotherapy*, *9*, 27–47.

Butnik, S. M. (2005). Neurofeedback in adolescents and adults with attention deficit hyperactivity disorder. *Journal of Clinical Psychology*, *61*, 621–625.

Callaway, T. G. & Bodenhamer-Davis, E. (2008). Long-term follow-up of a clinical replication of the Peniston Protocol for chemical dependency. *Journal of Neurotherapy*, *12* (4), 243 – 259.

Carmody, D. P., Radvanski, D. C., Wadhwani, S., Sabo, M. J. & Vergara, L. (2001). EEG biofeedback training and attention deficit/hyperactivity disorder in an elementary school setting. *Journal of Neurotherapy*, *4*, 5–27.

Chambers, J. C., Eccleston, L., Day, A., Ward, A. & Howells, K. (2008). Treatment readiness in violent offenders: The influence of cognitive factors on engagement in violence programs. *Aggression and Violent Behavior*, *13*, 276–284.

Craissati, J., South, R. & Bierer, K. (2009). Exploring the effectiveness of community sex offender treatment in relation to risk and re-offending. *The Journal of Forensic Psychiatry & Psychology*, *20*, 769–784.

Demos, J. N. (2005). *Getting started with neurofeedback*. New York: W.W. Norton & Company.

Dutton, D. G. (2006). *Rethinking domestic violence*. Vancouver, BC: UBC Press.

Engelbrecht, H. J., Kok, G., Vis, R., Keeser, D. & Deijen, J. B. (2010). Instrumentele conditionering van frontaalkwabactiviteit bij gezonde jongvolwassenen: Een dubbelblind placebogecontroleerd onderzoek naar EEG-neurofeedback. [Instrumental conditioning of frontal lobe activity in healthy young adults: A double-blind placebo-controlled study of EEG neurofeedback.] *Tijdschrift voor Neuropsychologie*, *1*, 16–26.

Evans, J. R. & Arbarbanel, A. (Eds.). (1999). *Introduction to quantitative EEG and neurofeedback*. San Diego, CA: Academic Press.

Fenger, T. N. (1998). Visual-motor integration and its relation to EEG neurofeedback brain wave patterns, reading, spelling, and arithmetic achievement in attention deficit disordered and learning disabled students. *Journal of Neurotherapy*, *2*, 9–18.

Fernández, T., Herrera, W., Harmony, T., Díaz-Comas, L., Santiago, E., Sánchez, L., Bosch, J., Fernández-Bouzas, A., Otero, G., Ricardo-Garcell, J., Barraza, C., Aubert, E., Galán, L. & Valdés, R. (2003). EEG and behavioral changes following neurofeedback treatment in learning disabled children. *Clinical EEG*, *34*, 3, 145-152.

Fuchs, T., Birbaumer, N., Lutzenberger, W., Gruzelier, J. H. & Kaiser, J. (2003). Neurofeedback treatment for attention-deficit/hyperactivity disorder in children: A comparison with methylphenidate. *Applied Psychophysiology & Biofeedback*, *28*, 1–12.

Glass, I. B. (1991). *The international handbook of addiction behaviour.* London: Routledge.

Gondolf, E. (1997). Patterns of reassault in batterer programs. *Violence and Victims, 12,* 338–349.

Gordon, J. A. & Moriarty, L. J. (2003). The effects of domestic violence batterer treatment on domestic violence recidivism. *Criminal Justice and Behavior, 30,* 103–110.

Gruzelier, J. & Egner, T. (2005). Critical validation studies of neurofeedback. *Child and Adolescent Psychiatric Clinics of North America, 14,* 83–104.

Hamel, J. & Nicholls, T. L. (2007). *Family interventions in domestic violence: A handbook of gender-inclusive theory and treatment.* New York, NY: Springer.

Hammond, D. C. (2003). QEEG-guided neurofeedback in the treatment of obsessive compulsive disorder. *The Journal of Neurotherapy, 7,* 25–52.

Hammond, D. C. (2007). What is Neurofeedback? *Journal of Neurotherapy, 10,* 4, 25-36.

Hampton, R. L., Gullotta, T. P. & Ramos, J. M. (2006). *Interpersonal violence in the African American community: Evidence-based prevention and treatment practices.* New York, NY: Springer.

Hanson, R. K., Gordon, A., Harris, A. J. R., Marques, J. K., Murphy, W., Quinsey, V. L. & Seto, M. C. (2002). First report of the collaborative outcome data project on the effectiveness of psychological treatment for sex offenders. *Sexual Abuse: A Journal of Research and Treatment, 14,* 169–194.

Hanson, R. K., Morton, K. E. & Harris, A. J. R. (2003). Sexual offender recidivism risk: What we know and what we need to know. *Annals of the New York Academy of Sciences, 989,* 154–166.

Heinrich, H., Gevensleben, H., Freisleder, F. J., Moll, G. H. & Rothenberger, A. (2004). Training of slow cortical potentials in attention-deficit/hyperactivity disorder: Evidence for positive behavioral and neurophysiological effects. *Biological Psychiatry, 55,* 772–775.

Jackson, N. A. (2007). *Encyclopedia of domestic violence*. New York, NY: Routledge.

Kaiser, D. A. & Othmer, S. (2000). Effect of neurofeedback on variables of attention in a large multi-center trial. *Journal of Neurotherapy*, *4*, 5–15.

Kelley, M. J. (1997). Native Americans, neurofeedback, and substance abuse theory: Three year outcome of alpha/theta neurofeedback training in the treatment of problem drinking among Dine' (Navajo) people. *Journal of Neurotherapy*, *2*, 24–60.

Kohl, P. L. & Macy, R. J. (2008). Profiles of victimized women among the child welfare population: Implications for targeted child welfare policy and practices. *Journal of Family Violence*, *23*, 57–68.

Kouijzer, M. E. J., De Moor, J. M. H., Gerrits, B. J. L., Buitelaar, J. K. & Van Schie, H. T. (2008). Long-term effects of neurofeedback treatment in autism. *Research in Autism Spectrum Disorders*. doi:1016/j.rasd.2008.10.003.

Kwan, G. (2002). Play attention! Can custom-made video games help kids with attention deficit disorder? *Berkeley Medical Journal*, Issues, *1*, 1–3.

Lin, S. C., Su, C. Y., Chou, F. H. C., Chen, S. P., Huang, J. J., Wu, G. T. E. & Chen, C. C. (2009). Domestic violence recidivism in high-risk Taiwanese offenders after the completion of violence treatment programs. *The Journal of Forensic Psychiatry & Psychology*, *20*, 458–472.

Linden, M., Habib, T. & Radojevic, V. (1996). A controlled study of the effects of EEG biofeedback on cognition and behaviour of children with attention deficit disorder and learning disabilities. *Biofeedback & Self Regulation*, *21*, 35–51.

Loeber, R., Slot, N. W. & Sergeant, J. A. (2001). *Ernstige en Gewelddadige Jeugddelinquentie: Omvang, oorzaken en interventies.* [*Serious and Violent Youth Delinquency: Size, causes and interventions.*] Houten/Diegem: Bohn Stafleu Van Loghum.

Lubar, J. F. & Lubar, J. O. (1999). Neurofeedback assessment and treatment for attention deficit/hyperactivity disorders. In R. Evans &

A. Arbarbanel (Eds.), *Introduction to quantitative EEG and neurofeedback*, (pp. 103–143). San Diego, CA: Academic Press.

Macy, R. J., Giattina, M. C., Parish, S. L. & Crosby, C. (2010). Domestic violence and sexual assault services: Historical concerns and contemporary challenges. *Journal of Interpersonal Violence, 25*, 3–32.

Marshall, W. L., Anderson, D. & Fernandez, Y. (1999). *Cognitive behavioural treatment of sexual offenders*. Chichester: Wiley.

Martin, G. & Johnson, C. L. (2005). The boys Totem town neurofeedback project: A pilot study of EEG biofeedback with incarcerated juvenile felons. *Journal of Neurotherapy, 9*, 71–86.

Masterpasqual, F. & Healey, K. N. (2003). Neurofeedback in psychological practice. *Professional Psychology: Research & Practice, 34*, 625–656.

McCue, M. L. (2008). *Domestic violence: A reference handbook*. 2nd ed. Santa Barbara, CA: ABC-CLIO.

McKay, J., Atterman, A., Rutherford, M., Cacciola, J. & McLellan, A. (1999). The relationship of alcohol use to cocaine relapse in cocaine dependent patients in an aftercare study. *Journal of Studies in Alcoholism, 60*, 176–180.

McKnight, J. Y. & Fehmi, L. G. (2001). Attention and neurofeedback synchrony training: Clinical results and their significance. *Journal of Neurotherapy, 5*, 45–61.

Miner, M. (2002). Factors associated with recidivism in juveniles: An analysis of serious juvenile sex offenders. *Journal of Research in Crime and Delinquency, 39*, 677–689.

Monastra, V. J., Lynn, S., Linden, M., Lubar, J. F., Gruzelier, J. & La Vaque, T. J. (2005). Electroencephalographic biofeedback in the treatment of attention deficit/hyperactivity disorder. *Journal of Neurotherapy, 9*, 5–34.

Monastra, V. J., Monastra, D. M. & George, S. (2002). The effects of stimulant therapy, EEG biofeedback and parenting style on the primary symptoms of attention deficit/hyperactivity disorder. *Applied Psychophysiology & Biofeedback, 27*, 231–249.

Nash, J. J. (2000). Treatment of attention deficit/hyperactivity disorder with neurotherapy. *Clinical Electroencephalography, 31*, 30–37.

Nestor, P. G. (2002). Mental disorder and violence: Personality dimensions and clinical features. *American Journal of Psychiatry, 159*, 1973–1978.

Othmer, S., Othmer, S. F. & Kaiser, D. A. (1999). EEG biofeedback: An emerging model for its global efficacy. In R. Evans & A. Arbarbanel (Eds.), *Introduction to quantitative EEG and neurofeedback*, (pp. 243–310). San Diego, CA: Academic Press.

Patrick, G. J. (1996). Improved neuronal regulation in ADHD: An application of fifteen sessions of photic-driven EEG neurotherapy. *Journal of Neurotherapy, 1*, 27–36.

Peek, W. H. M. & Nugter, M. A. (2009). Ik zit mijn tijd wel uit. . . Forensisch psychiatrische pilotstudie naar recidive bij patiënten met een strafrechtelijke plaatsing. [English summary: I'll serve my time . . . . A pilot study on recidivism in forensic patients forcibly hospitalized and treated for one year and on factors which affect recidivism]. *Tijdschrift voor Psychiatrie, 51*, 715–725.

Peniston, E. G. & Kulkoski, P. J. (1991). Alpha-theta brainwave neurofeedback for Vietnam veterans with combat-related post-traumatic stress disorder. *Medical Psychotherapy, 4*, 1–14.

Peniston, E. G. & Kulkoski, P. J. (1999). Neurofeedback in the treatment of addictive disorders. In J. R. Evans & A. Arbarbanel (Eds.), *Introduction to quantitative EEG and neurofeedback*, (pp. 157–179). San Diego, CA: Academic Press.

Peniston, E. G., Marrinan, D. A., Deming, W. A. & Kulcoski, P. J. (1993). EEG alpha-theta brainwave synchronization in Vietnam veterans with combat-related post traumatic stress disorder and alcohol abuse. *Advances in Medical Psychotherapy, 6*, 37-40.

Peterson, J. M. (2000). Notes on the role of neurotherapy in the treatment of posttraumatic stress disorder. *Biofeedback, 28*, 10–12.

Plichta, S. B. & Falik, M. (2001). Prevalence of violence and its implications for women's health. *Women's Health*, Issues 11, 244–258.

Quinn, J. F., Bodenhamer-Davis, E. & Koch, D. S. (2004). Ideology and the stagnation of AODA treatment modalities in America. *Deviant Behavior*, *25*, 109–131.

Robbins, J. (2000). *A symphony in the brain*. New York: Atlantic Monthly Press.

Rossiter, T. R. & La Vaque, T. J. (1995). A comparison of EEG biofeedback and psychostimulants in treating attention deficit hyperactivity disorders. *Journal of Neurotherapy*, *1*, 48–59.

Ryan, G. & Lane, S. (1997). *Juvenile sexual offending: Causes, consequences, and corrections*. San Francisco: Jossey-Bass Publishers.

Schulenburg, N. P. (1999). Neurofeedback therapy for ADHD and related neurological disorders. *Journal of Neurotherapy*, *3*, 10–20.

Scott, W., Brod, T. M., Siderof, S., Kaiser, D. & Sagan, M. (2002). *Type-specific EEG biofeedback improves residential substance abuse treatment*. Poster presentation at the meeting of the American Psychiatric Association, Philadelphia. Retrieved from http.//members. aol.com/williamscott/research.htm.

Scott, W., Kaiser, D., Othmer, S. & Sideroff, S. (2005). Effects of an EEG Biofeedback Protocol on a Mixed Substance Abusing Population. *American Journal of Alcohol and Drug Abuse*, *31*, 3, 455 – 469.

Seager, J., Jellicoe, D. & Dhaliwal, G. (2004). Refusers, dropouts, and completers: Measuring sex offender treatment efficacy. *International Journal of Offender Therapy and Comparative Criminology*, *48*, 600–612.

Smith, P. N. & Sams, M. W. (2005). Neurofeedback with juvenile offenders: A pilot study in the use of QEEG-based and analog-based remedial neurofeedback training. *Journal of Neurotherapy*, *9*, 87–99.

Sokhadze, E. M., Cannon, R. L. & Trudeau, D. L. (2008). EEG biofeedback as a treatment for Substance Use Disorders: review, rating of efficacy, and recommendations for further research. *Journal of Neurotherapy*, *12*(1), 5- 43.

Tansey, M. A. (1991). Wechsler (WISC-R) changes following treatment of learning disabilities via EEG biofeedback training in a private practice setting. *Australian Journal of Psychology*, *43*, 147–153.

't Hart-Kerkhoffs, L. A. (2010). *Juvenile sex offenders: Mental health and reoffending*. Amsterdam: Department of Child and Adolescent Psychiatry, VU University Medical Center.

Thompson, L. & Thompson, M. (1998). Neurofeedback combined with training in metacognitive strategies: Effectiveness in students with ADD. *Applied Psychophysiology & Biofeedback, 23*, 243–263.

Tinius, T. P. & Tinius, K. A. (2000). Changes after EEG biofeedback and cognitive retraining in adults with mild traumatic brain injury and attention deficit hyperactivity disorder. *Journal of Neurotherapy, 4*, 27–44.

Trudeau, D. L. (2000). The treatment of addictive disorders by brain wave biofeedback: A review and suggestions for future research. *Clinical Electroencephalography, 31*, 13–22.

Van Outsem, R. E. (2001). *De Aanpak: Systeemgerichte Hulp bij geweld in relaties*. Utrecht: Transact. [*The Approach: System-oriented Help with violence in relationships.*]

Van Outsem, R. E. (2009). *Exploring psychological characteristics of sexually abusive juveniles*. Utrecht: Forum Educatief.

Van Outsem, R. E. (2011). The applicability of neurofeedback in forensic psychotherapy: a literature review. *Journal of Forensic Psychiatry and Psychology, 22*, 2, 223-242.

Van Wijk, A. Ph. (2005). *Juvenile sex offenders and non-sex offenders: A comparative study*. Amsterdam: VU University.

Van Wijk, A. Ph., Bullens, R. A. R. & Van den Eshof, P. (2007). *Facetten van Zedencriminaliteit*. s-Gravenhage: Elsevier. [*Facets of Sex Crime.*]

Vermeiren, R. (2002). *Delinquents disordered? Psychopathology and neuropsychological deficits in delinquent adolescents*. Antwerp: Universiteit Antwerpen.

Vernon, D., Frick, A. & Gruzelier, J. (2004). Neurofeedback as a treatment for ADHD: A methodological review with implications for future research. *Journal of Neurotherapy, 8*, 53–82.

Welldon, E. V. & Van Velsen, C. (1996). *A practical guide to forensic psychotherapy*. London: Jessica Kingsley.

Wekerle, C. & Wall, A. M. (2002). *The violence and addiction equation: Theoretical and clinical issues in substance abuse and relationship violence*. New York, NY: Taylor & Francis.

Wijers, I. (2008). *Justitiële interventies voor jeugdige daders en risicojongeren*. [*Mandatory interventions for juvenile delinquents and for juveniles who are at risk of becoming delinquent*]. Den Haag: Boom Juridische Uitgevers.

Wilson, S. & Cumming, I. (2009). *Psychiatry in prisons*. Philadelphia, PA: Jessica Kingsleys.

In: Neurofeedback
Editor: Michael C. Hellinger

ISBN: 978-1-53615-167-1
© 2019 Nova Science Publishers, Inc.

Chapter 2

EEG-BASED LOCAL BRAIN ACTIVITY NEUROFEEDBACK (EEG-LBA-NF) – A NEW APPROACH IN TARGETING LOCALIZED REGIONS OF TRAINING

Herbert Bauer[1], Marleen Kempkes[1], Niels Birbaumer[2] and Ulrich Ansorge[1]

[1]Faculty of Psychology, University of Vienna, Vienna, Austria
[2]Medical Faculty, University of Tübingen, Tübingen, Germany
Wyss Center of Bio- and Neuroengineering, Geneva, Switzerland

ABSTRACT

In order to accomplish a targeted impact of neurofeedback on specific cortical functions 'EEG-based local brain activity neurofeedback training' (EEG-LBA-NF) was developed by Bauer et al., (2011). With this approach an implemented algorithm automatically identifies and localizes EEG-sources in successive sLORETA solutions. Based on this information the feedback is exclusively controlled by EEG-generating sources within a selected cortical region of training (ROT): Positive feedback is given if a source is located in the ROT and suspended if no source is detectable in the selected area. In this way the influence of sources in the vicinity of the ROT is excluded. In order to individually and precisely locate and define the ROT the use of evoked potentials (EPs) of known local origin is described and recommended. In addition to an evaluation via behavioral effects, this approach also enables the determination of the specificity of individual neurofeedback-applications on a neurophysiological level. First applications in both the time- and the frequency-domain yielded promising results: Subjects were able to significantly increase the feedback rate whereas controls receiving sham feedback were not.

Keywords: tomographic neurofeedback (tNF), EEG-LBA-NF, sLORETA

INTRODUCTION

In classical neurofeedback (NF) protocols single- or few-channel EEG-recordings are used. This procedure has the major limitation that the signal picked up by a single electrode is spatially unspecific: the electrical potential may be generated by sources close to the electrode or by more distant brain structures. Nunez et al. (1997) already described a simulation, estimating the distance of contributing sources to the measured scalp potential. The simulation was composed of three concentric spherical surfaces representing brain, skull and scalp. The sources were implemented as radial dipoles with fixed strength and were assumed to be uniformly distributed over the inner surface. The simulation predicted that about half of the contribution to the scalp potential derives from sources within a 3 cm radius around the recording electrode and more than 95% of the measured potential is generated by sources within a 6 cm surrounding. Even though the influence of spatially distributed sources in actual EEG recordings might differ from this simulation, the results indicate that single electrodes might pick up signals from relatively wide spread brain areas.

Therefore, using single electrodes for neurofeedback training poses the problem that the region generating a particular scalp signal is not known precisely and the region of training (ROT) is spatially undefined. Moreover, different participants might use different strategies, depending on which change of brain activity was first reinforced by positive feedback.

However, most studies on NF seem to disregard the question of *where* in the participants' brain the physiological changes occur and focus on the therapeutic outcome of the training. The therapeutic outcome is commonly assessed via introspection and/or on the behavioral level. These measurements may on the one hand produce false positive results as NF can produce unspecific (placebo) effects (Schabus et al, 2017; Liechti et al., 2012) and on the other hand false negative results, as some participants may not experience any therapeutic relief if they weren't able to change their brain activity (Alkoby et al., 2018). Hence, more placebo controlled NF studies are needed in which the ROT will be targeted precisely and therefore a possible therapeutic outcome could be ascribed to the physiological changes in circumscribed brain areas leading to further testable hypotheses about the mechanisms underlying neurofeedback.

Attempts to Improve the Spatial Specificity of NF Training

Efforts to improve the spatial specificity of NF training have been stimulated by the growing availability of tomographic brain activity recording techniques.

Aside to the development of real time functional magnetic resonance tomography neurofeedback (rtfMRT-NF) (Posse et al., 2003; Weiskopf et al., 2003; deCharms et al., 2004; Sitaram, et al., 2011; Weiskopf, 2012; Birbaumer, et al., 2013; Thibault, et al., 2016; Watanabe, et al., 2017) and near infrared spectroscopy neurofeedback (NIRS-NF) (Mihara et al., 2012; Kober et al., 2014; Ehlis et al., 2018), electromagnetic tomographic techniques have been proposed. Applications of rtfMRI-NF showed promising results by successfully enhancing the BOLD activity in targeted structures, which had an impact on the whole functional network the structure is part of (Zotev et al., 2018).

In the field of electromagnetic imaging, soon after the publication of LORETA, a distributed source modelling algorithm for localizing sources of multi-channel time or frequency domain EEG/MEG-signals using a three-shell spherical head model (Pascual Marqui et al., 1994), M.

Congedo developed a real-time variant for NF-applications called 'tomographic NF (tNF)' – also 'LORETA neurofeedback (LNFB)' (Congedo et al., 2004). With this first EEG-based tomographic NF procedure the feedback signal mirrors directly the estimated current density values of voxels selected from the solution space as region of training (ROT). The behavioral and cognitive outcome and the impact on EEG characteristics of this frequency domain LNFB, as proposed by Congedo et al., (2004), have been investigated by R. Cannon and coworkers in several studies yielding varying degrees of success (Cannon et al., 2006, 2007, 2008, 2009, 2014). Astonishingly, the more advanced method, 'sLORETA,' also developed by Pascual Marqui and published in 2002, which employs a realistic head model was not utilized in these studies.

sLORETA-NF was applied only recently in a study of 13 children diagnosed with ADHD by Liechti et al., (2012). This study used EEG frequency as well as slow cortical potential (SCP) signal components and a single voxel within the anterior cingulate cortex (ACC) as 'ROT.' Quite informative, especially on more general aspects of NF, no learning in the ACC was observed but therapeutic effects were in the usual range of NF studies – maybe due to the very strict regime to avoid EEG signal artifacts; this regime had a significant effect on artifact reduction but may also have acted as a behavioral intervention. Positive sLORETA-NF results have been reported in a study targeting the left hemispheric linguistic areas – results are discussed below in section "first applications" (Bauer et. al, 2011).

sLORETA-NF software, which utilizes EEG signals from only 19 electrodes placed according to the international 10/20 system, is now commercially available and has already found its way into psychiatric institutions and psychotherapist's offices (see Thacher and Lubar, 2014). In this context, however, it needs to be strongly emphasized that true spatial specificity of feedback is only achievable when following basic rules of digital signal processing as well as keeping performance limits of algorithms for invers solutions in mind. It should be emphasized that only restricted information on the generating 3-dimensional neuronal activity pattern within the cortex is accessible via scalp potential distributions. As a consequence, sLORETA estimates are strongly shaped by the invers procedure, yield highly correlated spatially neighboring values (spatial blurring) and do not exactly mirror the real generating current density (CD) distribution. Therefore, compared with traditional NF, sLORETA-NF that simply mirrors back sLORETA estimates of single voxels or groups of voxels would not be much more spatially specific.

EEG-BASED LBA-NEUROFEEDBACK (EEG-LBA-NF) TRAINING

Instrumental learning, NF's core mechanism of action, requires correct and consistent reinforcement during the ongoing learning process. As a consequence for targeted NF, all desired activity-changes directly generated by a particular cortical structure (i.e., the ROT) have to be reinforced (fed back) in order to achieve a durable modification of the activity in this selected structure. In most cases, however, scalp potential distributions are generated by several simultaneously active sources and possibly weaker sources in the ROT should not be missed for feedback. In order to enable the detection of simultaneously active sources, 'simultaneous multiple sources' (SMS-) LORETA was developed as the core procedure of EEG-based LBA-neurofeedback (EEG-LBA-NF).

Utilizing a 3-shell realistic head model the sLORETA algorithm basically transforms scalp potential distributions into standardized 3D CD distributions within the predefined solution space representing the cerebral cortex. SMS-LORETA has the additional feature of identifying all generator loci i.e., all local maxima, in such sLORETA solutions automatically (Pllana and Bauer, 2008, 2011).

SMS-LORETA is composed of

- an iterative loop: recorded scalp potential distribution > sLORETA transformation > storage of the maximum CD's spatial location > calculation of a forward solution i.e., surface potential distribution,

that corresponds to a standardized source at this location >
cumulative subtraction of this forward solution from the recorded
scalp potential distribution > as new input to sLORETA until the
initially recorded scalp potential distribution is flat; and
- a 'spatially sensitive' cluster analysis of all stored maximum CD
locations; and
- the identification of all cluster centers which then are taken as loci
of generating source with the maximum CD within each cluster as
their corresponding and estimated strength.

Following this procedure, a feedback program can automatically and
rapidly decide whether a source is present within the predefined ROT and
execute feedback accordingly.

FIRST APPLICATIONS OF EEG-LBA-NF

Pilot-sessions using this new feedback algorithm revealed quite low
feedback rates initially, which turned out to be insufficient to initiate
instrumental learning. These observations have led to an implementation in
which LBA-NF is executed trial-wise in a task-/stimulus-linked manner.
Via computer screen trainees are presented with short stimuli or tasks
(1–8s), which involve the ROT-structures to a variable extent. Trainees are
instructed to respond to these stimuli or tasks accordingly, and mentally
repeat these responses during the presentation period. Artifact and pre-
stimulus baseline corrected scalp potential distributions at selectable
latencies are extracted from the ongoing multi-channel EEG and analyzed
with SMS-LORETA. If this analysis identifies a source within the ROT, its
strength determines the brightness of a green frame around the
stimulus/task presentation area on the computer screen. If no source is
found within the ROT, the frame remains or turns gray. This feedback is
updated after each stimulus/task presentation according to the current
SMS-LORETA outcome. As a general instruction, trainees are asked to try
to keep the frame brightly green as long as possible.

In order to achieve sufficiently accurate source localization, adequate spatial sampling i.e., a sufficient number of electrodes distributed fairly equally across the scalp, is essential. According to the literature and to results of our own simulation studies, ideally around 60 but not less than 40 electrodes should be used (Shrinivasan, 1998; Freeman et al., 203; Lau et al., 2012; Pllana and Bauer, 2011). Spatial under-sampling causes spatial aliasing i.e., modifies the input topography, on the one hand and on the other hand impairs the precision of the sLORETA inverse solution.

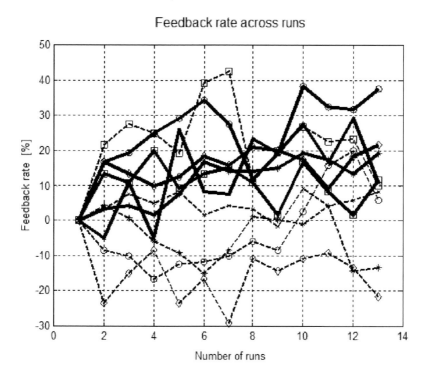

Figure 1. Feedback for focal activity in the left-hemispheric linguistic areas. Individual course of the feedback rate across runs separated for subjects in the experimental group (solid lines) and the control group (dashed lines).

A first study aimed to explore the feasibility of this new EEG-LBA-NF algorithm; it investigated whether subjects are able to learn to increase the activity within their left-hemispheric linguistic areas (ROT; BA 6, 21, 22, 40, 44, 45) by means of the task-linked procedure (Bauer et al., 2011). Ten healthy right-handed subjects participated in daily training sessions on seven consecutive days. Five of them received consistent feedback (experimental group; EG) the other five sham feedback (control group; CG). Daily sessions had two runs of 120 item presentations each. The last run was a transfer trial, in which the participants did not receive any feedback. They were asked to behave as they did in the run before. Items were sketches of simple actions, each presented on a computer screen for 3 s with varying inter-stimulus intervals of 6 +/- 2 s. Subjects were asked to covertly name the verb that corresponded to the presented item and, concurrently, to turn the gray frame around the item presentation area as intensively green as possible. Simultaneous to the item presentation 58-channel DC-EEG signal epochs were recorded and SMS-LORETA analyzed at three latencies. EG-members received feedback as a green frame whenever generating sources were detected in the ROT, CG-members got green feedback randomly at a rate of 20% of the items per run, but with hidden online SMS-LORETA analyses (for details see Bauer et al., 2011; Bauer and Pllana, 2014). Taking the average number of 'within-ROT sources' per run as a measure of the NF learning process, an increase across the runs was observed in the EG but not in the CG – see Figure 1. This difference was statistically significant (Man-Whitney U test; $p < .01$).

Furthermore, an ongoing project aims to evaluate the feasibility of frequency-domain LBA-NF. Conceptualized as a possible therapy of tinnitus, this first implementation aims to facilitate and enhance EEG-alpha activity in the auditory cortices. Again, training sessions are designed in a trial-wise manner (two runs of 50 trials each) with noise presentation and a dark computer screen during the inter-trial intervals. With the beginning of each 15 s trial (training phase) the noise will be interrupted and a rectangular window opens up on the screen and delayed by 1 s small narrow gray bars appear from left to right in steps of 200 ms reaching the right end of the window after 15 s. Concurrently with the 200-ms-steps the preceding 58-channel EEG-signal epochs of 1 s duration are extracted, eye movement artifact corrected and analyzed by the frequency domain variant of SMS-LORETA. Whenever a source within the frequency range of 10 to

12 Hz is detected, the corresponding gray bar turns green and becomes bigger mirroring the strength of the source as a feedback. Subjects' task is to make as many gray bars as possible green and bigger.

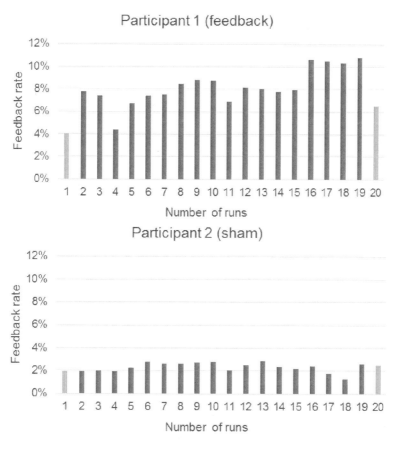

Figure 2: Preliminary experimental outcome. Feedback rate for one participant (1) receiving EEG-LBA-NF to enhance alpha activity in the left auditory cortex and a second participant (2) receiving sham feedback. The training was carried out over ten consecutive days with two runs per day. The first and last run were transfer trails without feedback.

Before using this new NF procedure with tinnitus patients, screening runs with healthy participants are performed in order to evaluate the feasibility of this implantation. In Figure 2 the results of one experimental and one control subject are shown as examples. Taking the number of 'within-ROT sources' as a measure of learning, a clear increase appears across runs for the experimental but not for the control subject.

CONCLUSION

These first and preliminary observations demonstrate that subjects are able to modify their cortical activity spatially targeted by means of EEG-LBA-NF and, are encouraging for continuing this line of research in the following respects:

1. Whether the application of EEG-LBA-NF leads to long-lasting changes on the physiological, behavioral, and cognitive level is to be shown by future research.
2. Since the frequency domain EEG-LBA-NF design as described above seems to be efficient it suggests its application also with time domain signals – thus creating a spatially sensitive version of slow cortical potential (SCP-) NF.
3. Evaluation of possible advantages of utilizing beamforming filters in the SMS-procedure instead of sLORETA may lead to less blurry 3D estimates of the source power throughout the cerebral cortex (VanVeen et al., 1997; Greenand and McDonald, 2009; Grosse-Wentrup et al., 2009).
4. Being aware of the limited accuracy and spatial resolution of sLORETA, however, a kind of calibration procedure is indispensable for the purposes of personalizing the head model's topography of cortical areas within the solution space. As a first attempt, sLORETA localized generators of particular evoked potentials (EP) may be used with sensory and motor areas to adjust the ROT individually. For example, the auditory steady state response (ASSR) is appropriate to determine the individual location of the primary auditory cortices within the solution space. Within frontal areas it is more difficile because EP components with accurately known origin in the frontal cortex are sparse –

error-related negativity (ERN), feedback-related negativity (FRN), perhaps. Anyway, 'personalizing the head model's topography of cortical structures/functions' has the advantage that additional to the individually varying head geometries all inherent inaccuracies of the simplifying bio-physical model used with source localization procedures would be taken into consideration and compensated for.

ACKNOWLEDGMENTS

The developments of the EEG-LBA-NF training over the years was supported by grant #12475 (Austria National Bank) and grant #P19830-B02 (Austrian Science Fund, FWF). The development of the frequency domain EEG-LBA-NF was supported by grant number #290833054 (German Research Foundation, Deutsche Forschungsgemeinschaft, DFG).

REFERENCES

Alkoby, O., Abu-Rmileh, A., Shriki, O. & Todder, D. (2018). Can we predict who will respond to neurofeedback? A review of the inefficacy problem and existing predictors for successful EEG neurofeedback learning. *Neuroscience* 378, 155-164.

Bauer, H., Pllana, A. and Sailer, U. (2011). The EEG-based local brain activity (LBA-) feedback training. *Act. Nerv. Super Rediviva* 53, 107–113.

Bauer H., Pllana A. (2014). EEG-based local brain activity feedback training—tomographic neurofeedback. *Frontiers in Human Neuroscience*, Perspective article: Vol. 8, Article 1005. doi: 10.3389/fnhum.2014.01005.

Birbaumer, N. et al., (2013). Learned regulation of brain metabolism. *Trends Cogn. Sci.* 17, 295–302.

Cannon, R. L., Baldwin, D. R., Diloreto, D. J., Phillips, S. T., Shaw, T. L. and Levy, J. J. (2014). LORETA neurofeedback in the precuneus: operant conditioning in basic mechanisms of self-regulation. *Clin. EEG Neurosci.* 45, 238–248. doi:10. 1177/1550059413512796.

Cannon, R., Congedo, M., Lubar, J. F., and Hutchens, T. (2009). Differentiating a network of executive attention: LORETA neurofeedback in anterior cingulate and dorsolateral prefrontal cortices. *Int. J. Neurosci.* 119, 404–441. doi:10. 1080/0020745080 2480325.

Cannon, R., Lubar, J. F., Congedo, M., Thornton, K., Towler, K. and Hutchens, T. (2007). The effect of neurofeedback training in the cognitive division of the anterior cingulate gyrus. *Int. J. Neurosci.* 117, 337–357. doi:10. 1080/00207450500514003.

Cannon, R., Lubar, J. F., Gerke, A., Thornton, K., Hutchens, T. and McCammon, V. (2006). EEG spectral-power and coherence: LORETA neurofeedback training in the anterior cingulate gyrus. *J. Neurother.* 10, 5–31. doi:10.1300/j184v10n01_02.

Cannon, R., Lubar, J. F., Sokhadze, E. and Baldwin, D. R. (2008). LORETA neurofeedback for addiction and the possible neurophysiology of psychological processes influenced: a case study and region of interest analysis of LORETA neurofeedback in right anterior cingulate cortex. *J. Neurother.* 12, 227–241. doi:10.1080/ 10874200802501948.

Congedo, M., Lubar, J. F. and Joffe, D. (2004). Low-resolution electromagnetic tomography neurofeedback. *IEEE Trans. Neural. Syst. Rehabil. Eng.* 12, 387–397. doi:10.1109/tnsre.2004.840492.

deCharms, R. C., Christoff, K., Glover, G.H., Pauly, J. M., Whitfield, S. and Gabrieli, J. D. (2004). Learned regulation of spatially localized brain activation using real-time fMRI. *Neuroimage* 21, 436–443. doi:10.1016/j.neuroimage.2003.08.041.

Ehlis, A-Ch., Barth, B., Hudak, J., Storchak, H., Weber, L., Kimmig, A-Ch. S., Kreifelts, B., Dresler, Th. and Fallgatter A. J. (2018). Near-Infrared Spectroscopy as a new Tool for Neurofeedback Training:

Applications in Psychiatry and Methodological Considerations. *Japanese Psychological Association*. doi: 10.1111/jpr.12225.

Freeman, W. J., Holmes, M. D., Burke, B.C. and Vanhatalo, S. (2003). Spatial Spectra of scalp EEG and EMG from awake humans. *Clin. Neurophysiol*. 114, 1053–1068. doi:10.1016/s1388-2457(03)00045-2.

Green, J. J. and McDonald, J. J. (2009). A practical guide to beamformer source reconstruction for EEG, In: T. C. Handy (Ed), *Brain Signal Analysis: Advances in Neuroelectric and Neuromagnetic Methods,* (Cambridge, MA: The MITPress), 79–98.

Grosse-Wentrup, M., Liefhold, C., Gramann, K. and Buss, M. (2009). Beamforming in non-invasive brain-computer interfaces. *IEEE Trans. Biomed. Eng*. 56, 1209–1219. doi:10.1109/tbme.2008.2009768.

Kober, S. E., Wood, G., Kurzmann, J., Friedrich, E. V. C., Stangl, M., Wippel, T., et al., (2014). Near-infrared spectroscopy based neurofeedback training increases specific motor imagery related cortical activation compared to sham feedback. *Biol. Psychol*. 95, 21–30.doi:10.1016/j.biopsycho.2013.05.005.

Lau, TM, Gwin, JT, Ferris, DP. (2012) How Many Electrodes Are Really Needed for EEG-Based Mobile Brain Imaging? *Journal of Behavioral and Brain Science,* 2012, 2, 387-393.

Liechti, M. D., Maurizio, S., Heinrich, H., Jäncke, L., Meier, L., Steinhausen, H-C., et al., (2012). First clinical trial of tomographic neurofeedback in attention-deficit/ hyperactivity disorder: evaluation of voluntary cortical control. *Clin. Neurophysiol*. 123, 1989–2005. doi:10.1016/j.clinph.2012.03.016.

Mihara, M., Miyai, I., Hattori, N., Hatakenaka, M., Yagura, H., Kawano, T., et al., (2012). Neurofeedback using real-time near-infrared spectroscopy enhances motor imagery related cortical activation. *PloS One* 7:e32234. doi:10.1371/journal.pone.0032234.

Nunez, P. L., Srinivasan, R., Westdorp, A. F., Wijesinghe, R. S., Tucker, D. M., Silberstein, R. B., & Cadusch, P. J. (1997). EEG coherency: I: statistics, reference electrode, volume conduction, Laplacians, cortical imaging, and interpretation at multiple scales. *Electroencephalography and clinical neurophysiology*, 103(5), 499-515.

Pascual-Marqui, R. D. (2002). Standardized low resolution brain electromagnetic tomography (sLORETA): technical details. *Methods Find Exp. Clin. Pharmacol.* 24 D, 5–12.

Pascual-Marqui, R. D., Michel, C. M. and Lehmann, D. (1994). Low resolution electromagnetic tomography: a new method for localizing electrical activity in the brain. *Int. J. Psychophysiol.* 18, 49–65. doi:10.1016/0167-8760(84)90014-x.

Pllana, A. and Bauer, H. (2008). Localization of simultaneous multiple sources using SMS-LORETA. *arXiv*: 2008; 0806.4845[q-bio], http://arxiv.org/ftp/arxiv/papers/0806/0806.4845.pdf.

Pllana, A. and Bauer, H. (2011). BEM-based SMS-LORETA an advanced method to localize multiple simultaneously active sources in the cerebral cortex. *arXiv*: 2011; http://arxiv.org/ftp/arxiv/papers/1106/ 1106.2679.pdf.

Posse, S., Fitzgerald, D., Gao, K., Habel, U., Rosenberg, D., Moore, G. J., et al., (2003). Real-time fMRI of temporo-limbic regions detects amygdala activation during single-trial self-induced sadness. *Neuroimage* 18, 760–768. doi:10. 1016/s1053-8119(03)00004-1.

Schabus, M., Griessenberger, H., Gnjezda, M. T., Heib, D. P., Wislowska, M., and Hoedlmoser, K. (2017). Better than sham? A double-blind placebo-controlled neurofeedback study in primary insomnia. *Brain*, 140 (2), 1-12. doi:10.1093/brain/awx011.

Sitaram, R., Lee, S., Ruiz, S. and Birbaumer, N. (2011). Real-time regulation and Detection of brain states from fMRI signals, in *Neurofeedback and Neuromodulation Techniques and Applications*, Eds Coben, R., and Evans, J. R. New York: Academic Press, pp.: 227– 249.

Srinivasan, R., Tucker, D. M. and Murias, M. (1998). Estimating the spatial Nyquist of the human EEG. *Behav. Res. Methods. Instrum. Comput.* 30, 8–19. doi:10. 3758/bf03209412.

Thatcher, R. W. and Lubar, J. F. (Eds.) (2014). *Z Score Neurofeedback: Clinical Applications.* Academic Press, San Diego, CA.

Thibault, R. T., Lifshitz, M., Raz, A. (2016). The self-regulating brain and neurofeedback: experimental science and clinical promise. *Cortex* 74, 247–261.

Van Veen, B. D., Van Drongelen, W., Yuchtman, M. and Suzuki, A. (1997). Localization of brain electrical activity via linearly constrained minimum variance spatial filtering. *IEEE Trans. Biomed. Eng.* 44, 867–880. doi:10.1109/10. 623056.

Watanabe, T., Sasaki, Y., Shibata, K. and Kawato, M. (2017). Advances in fMRI Real-Time Neurofeedback. *Trends in Cognitive Sciences*, 21: 12. http://dx.doi.org/10.1016/j.tics.2017.09.010.

Weiskopf, N. (2012). Real-time fMRI and its application to neurofeedback. *Neuroimage* 62, 682–692. doi:10.1016/j.neuroimage.2011.10.009.

Weiskopf, N., Veit, R., Erb, M., Mathiak, K., Grodd, W., Goebel, R., et al., (2003). Physiological self-regulation of regional brain activity using real-time functional magnetic resonance imaging (fMRI): methodology and exemplary data. *Neuroimage* 19, 577–586. doi:10.1016/s1053-8119(03)00145-9.

Zotev, V., Phillips, R., Misaki, M., Wong, Ch. K., Wurfel, B. E., Krueger, F., Feldner, M., Bodurka, J. (2018). Real-time fMRI neurofeedback training of the amygdala activity with simultaneous EEG in veterans with combat-related PTSD. *NeuroImage: Clinical* 19: 106 – 121.

In: Neurofeedback   ISBN: 978-1-53615-167-1
Editor: Michael C. Hellinger   © 2019 Nova Science Publishers, Inc.

Chapter 3

NEUROFEEDBACK TRAINING AND PHYSICAL TRAINING IMPACTED ON MOTOR SKILLS AMONG VETERANS WITH SPINAL CORD INJURY

Ebrahim Norouzi[1,] and Mohammad Vaezmosavi[2]*
[1]Department of Human Motor Behavior, Faculty of Physical Education and Sports, Urmia University, Urmia, Iran
[2]Department of Physical Education, Faculty of Social Sciences, Emam Hosien University, Tehran, Iran

ABSTRACT

Spinal cord injuries (SCIs) demand particular attention; people with SCI report reduced quality of life and impairments in everyday life. We tested whether and if so to what extent neurofeedback or a physical training could, compared to a control condition, improve reaction time and balance as proxies for fine motor control in a sample of Iranian veterans with SCI. A total of 30 Iranian veterans with SCI were randomly assigned to the following study conditions: neurofeedback, physical

---
* Corresponding Author Email: eb.norouzi@urmia.ac.ir. Address: Department of Motor Behavior, Faculty of Sport, Urmia University, Urmia, Iran.

training, or a control condition (conventional therapy). Both at the beginning and four weeks later, reaction times and balance were objectively measured. Compared to the control condition and over time, reaction times improved in the neurofeedback condition, while balance improved in the physical training condition. Compared to a conventional treatment condition, neurofeedback and physical training improved skills in specific areas of motor control. Thus, it appears that both neurofeedback and physical training should be introduced as routine interventions for patients with SCIs.

Keywords: motor performance, exercise training, rehabilitation, reaction time, balance, neurofeedback

INTRODUCTION

Spinal Cord Injuries (SCIs) are considered a serious health problem (Post & Noreau, 2005). Typically, adults with SCIs suffer from disorders of the cardiovascular and respiratory systems, along with chronic pain; they also report reduced quality of life. Thus, SCIs are associated with considerable reductions in functional status, including poor motor performance, and extensive psychological issues such as severe negative emotion and low self-esteem as well as increased needs for medical and paramedical support (Harvey, 2016). Prevalence rates have been estimated at between 50 to 1,298 cases per million population worldwide; the range varies considerably across occupations (Young, Webster, Giunti, Pransky, & Nesathurai, 2006). For example, the risk of injury involving SCIs is particularly high among construction industry workers (26%), transportation and retail workers (15% each), manufacturing workers (13%), and agriculture and utility workers (11% each), whereas some other occupations have a low risk of such injury (Eslami, Dehghan, & Rahimi-Movaghar, 2015). Additionally, and not surprisingly, prevalence rates for SCIs are high among soldiers, and this holds particularly true for those soldiers doing their service under wartime conditions.

Treatment options for SCIs include physical therapy, occupational therapy, and rehabilitation psychology, along with various forms of medication. These last are widely employed to treat pain and muscular spasms, though, they also have side-effects. In the present study, we focused on physical training (PT) and on neurofeedback.

While PT is well established as a treatment for SCIs, more recently neurofeedback (NF) and neurofeedback training (NFT) have attracted increased interest. For instance, NF and NFT have been employed to treat pain, as the feedback via the neurofeedback device serves to reinforce neuronal activities associated with specific brain activities (Sitaram et al., 2017). Within the field of NFT, a 12- to 15-Hz oscillation of the sensorimotor cortex has proved to be a promising link between adaptive mental states and skilled visuo-motor performance (Egner & Gruzelier, 2004). A 12- to 15-Hz oscillation of the sensorimotor cortex is also referred to as Sensorimotor Rhythm (SMR). There is now evidence of the positive effects of NFT in adults with chronic pain (Warms, Turner, Marshall, & Cardenas, 2002), attention-deficit/hyperactivity disorder (Strehl et al., 2006), and fibromyalgia (Caro & Winter, 2011) , with impacts on motor performance enhancement (Rayegani et al., 2014), and cognitive flexibility (Sitaram et al., 2017). Neurofeedback has also been employed in the treatment of anxiety and traumatic brain injury, and in the recovery of patients with impaired motor performance (Sitaram et al., 2017). Additionally, NFT has the potential to replace aspects of physical exercising, particularly among people with disabilities (Rayegani et al., 2014) and thus for whom regular participation in physical exercises could be rather difficult, while ameliorating health-related problems associated with a sedentary life style.

To summarize, both PT and NFT have the potential to improve motor control among people with SCIs, but surprisingly previous scientific efforts have focused primarily on pain relief. In this respect, it is important to emphasize that NFT does not have a negative impact on motor performance (Rayegani et al., 2014), or spinal cord lesions (Jensen et al., 2013). We believe that answers to these questions might help both caregivers and patients with SCI improve the latter's motor skills, which in turn could have positive effects on quality of life.

METHODS

Participants

At total of 30 Iranian low paraplegia veterans (SCI at L3, L4 (ASIA B - D) took part in the study. Mean age was 51.5 years (SD = 3.87), and mean weight was 82.0kg (SD = 8.94). Inclusion criteria were: 1) Iranian male veteran; 2) age between 48 and 60 years; 3) spinal cord injury and grade $\geq$ 3 of sensation according to the International Standards for Neurological Classification of SCI; 4) right handed (assessed by the Edinburgh Handedness Inventory; 5) signed written informed consent. Exclusion criteria were: 1) psychiatric issues, as ascertained by a brief psychiatric interview; 2) intake of mood- and alertness-altering medications or substances.

CONCLUSION

As the results indicated, NFT had greater influence than PT on upper extremity function patients with SCI. That can be due to the effect of psychological variables on upper limb reaction time like relaxing attention focus through which we can improve this variable with NFT. Therefore, it is recommended to use NFT for veterans' upper extremity motor recovery from spinal cord injuries.

Numerous studies have been conducted to examine the effect of physical therapy techniques to reduce intensified muscles and to improve balance and gait parameters that have some impacts on them and ineffective neurofeedback techniques have been assessed. Moreover, PT was more effective than NFT in improving balance of veterans with SCI. Because the control centers of vestibule are balanced, so the PT is more effective when the vestibular control factors are considered. Cawthorne and Cooksey exercises are training of vestibular rehabilitation exercises that balance control centers such as: vision, proprioception through which vestibular system is involved. According to the findings of existing studies and the results we can say that Cawthorne and Cooksey training may improve balance in the veterans with SCI and should restore the balance in the veterans' treatment with spinal cord injuries while it was unaware of these types of training.

REFERENCES

Caro, X. J., & Winter, E. F. (2011). EEG biofeedback treatment improves certain attention and somatic symptoms in fibromyalgia: a pilot study. *Appl. Psychophysiol. Biofeedback*, 36(3), 193-200. doi:10.1007/s 10484-011-9159-9.

Egner, T., & Gruzelier, J. H. (2004). EEG biofeedback of low beta band components: frequency-specific effects on variables of attention and event-related brain potentials. *Clin. Neurophysiol.*, 115(1), 131-139.

Eslami, V., Dehghan, F., & Rahimi-Movaghar, V. (2015). Dimensions of Quality of Life in Spinal Cord Injured Veterans of Iran: a Qualitative Study. *Acta Med. Iran*, 53(12), 753-763.

Harvey, L. A. (2016). Physiotherapy rehabilitation for people with spinal cord injuries. *J. Physiother.*, 62(1), 4-11. doi:10.1016/j.jphys. 2015.11.004.

Jensen, M. P., Gertz, K. J., Kupper, A. E., Braden, A. L., Howe, J. D., Hakimian, S., & Sherlin, L. H. (2013). Steps toward developing an EEG biofeedback treatment for chronic pain. *Appl. Psychophysiol. Biofeedback*, 38(2), 101-108. doi:10.1007/s10484-013-9214-9.

Post, M., & Noreau, L. (2005). Quality of life after spinal cord injury. *J. Neurol. Phys.Ther.*, 29(3), 139-146.

Rayegani, S. M., Raeissadat, S. A., Sedighipour, L., Rezazadeh, I. M., Bahrami, M. H., Eliaspour, D., & Khosrawi, S. (2014). Effect of neurofeedback and electromyographic-biofeedback therapy on improving hand function in stroke patients. Top Stroke Rehabil., 21(2), 137-151. doi:10.1310/tsr2102-137.

Sitaram, R., Ros, T., Stoeckel, L., Haller, S., Scharnowski, F., Lewis-Peacock, J., . . . Sulzer, J. (2017). Closed-loop brain training: the science of neurofeedback. *Nat. Rev. Neurosci.,* 18(2), 86-100. doi:10.1038/nrn.2016.164.

Strehl, U., Leins, U., Goth, G., Klinger, C., Hinterberger, T., & Birbaumer, N. (2006). Self-regulation of slow cortical potentials: a new treatment for children with attention-deficit/hyperactivity disorder. *Pediatrics,* 118(5), e1530-1540. doi:10.1542/peds.2005-2478.

Warms, C. A., Turner, J. A., Marshall, H. M., & Cardenas, D. D. (2002). Treatments for chronic pain associated with spinal cord injuries: many are tried, few are helpful. *Clin. J. Pain.,* 18(3), 154-163.

Young, A., Webster, B., Giunti, G., Pransky, G., & Nesathurai, S. (2006). Rehospitalization following compensable work-related tetraplegia. *Spinal Cord,* 44(6), 374-382. doi:10.1038/sj.sc.3101858.

In: Neurofeedback   ISBN: 978-1-53615-167-1
Editor: Michael C. Hellinger   © 2019 Nova Science Publishers, Inc.

Chapter 4

THE EFFECT OF NEUROFEEDBACK TRAINING ON SPORT PERFORMANCE AND CONSCIOUS MOTOR PROCESSING AMONG SKILLED DART PLAYERS

Ebrahim Norouzi[1,], Fatemehsadat Hosseini[1] and Mohammad Vaezmosavi[2]*

[1]Department of Human Motor Behavior, Faculty of Physical Education and Sports, Urmia University, Urmia, Iran
[2]Department of Physical Education, Faculty of Social Sciences, Emam Hosien University, Tehran, Iran

ABSTRACT

The use of neurofeedback is growing rapidly in sport performance enhancement. The aim of this study was to investigate the effect of neurofeedback training on motor performance and conscious motor processing of skilled dart players. The participants were 20 male skilled dart players. The research was conducted in five phases, include: Pre-test, training neurofeedback, posttest 1, under pressure test and posttest 2.

* Corresponding Author Email: eb.norouzi@urmia.ac.ir.

Training neurofeedback was consisted of prevent training to the Alpha band frequency (8 to 12 Hz) in F4. To data analyze descriptive statistics and Mixed ANOVA was used. Results indicate the amount of conscious motor processing for neurofeedback training group decreased at post-test 1($p = 0.001$) and, under pressure test. However, this reduction was not observed in the control group. The dart throw points for neurofeedback training group and control group in the post-test 1 compare to per-test were enhanced but only neurofeedback group($p = 0.001$) be able preserve this increase in the under pressure test. This study indicates, there are influences among neurofeedback training, conscious motor processing and athletic performance. In other words, the neurofeedback training by reducing the conscious motor processing leads to the desired motor performance and creates automatic sense in the athlete

Keywords: conscious processing, quiet mind, neurofeedback, dart throw, under pressure

INTRODUCTION

It is believed that physical training is created the changes in athletes, their muscles become strengthened, the amount of uptake oxygen increased, the technical skills are more efficient, and they are able to do more with less effort (Vickers, 2007). These biochemical and physiological changes are well-known, but positive brain changes such as optimal patterns of electroencephalographic (EEG) are less well-known in sport and exercise training. Achieving optimal performance requires proper mental conditions. Quantification of mental conditions during coaching is often a difficult task. With new tools such as the Neurofeedback, you can record and present athletic brain activity. The use of neurofeedback is growing rapidly in sport performance enhancement. Neurofeedback training (NFT) also leads to implicit learning. For example, alpha waves of 8 to 12 Hz in the F4 region are responsible for task-relevant explicit (declarative knowledge). By suppressing this frequency band, it can create the same conditions as implicit learning. The reduction of alpha at the F4 position reflects increased motor learning. Therefore, the aim of this study was to investigate the effect of neurofeedback training on motor performance and conscious motor processing of skilled dart players.

METHODS

Participants

The participant was not informed about the effect of the intervention, and in other words, the blind-approach research was conducted. This approach spoiled the expectation of the subject to reaching a high level of performance after the intervention. The participants were 20 male skilled dart players. The research was conducted in five phases, include: Pre-test, training neurofeedback, posttest 1, under pressure test and posttest 2. Pre-test: At this stage, the subjects performed 20 dart throwing attempts. Training: The subjects continued to practice for five days on their terms and protocols. On the first day of the training, the subjects performed two dart blocks of 20 attempts. 5 days of workout completed with 200 attempts. Training neurofeedback was consisted of prevent training to the Alpha band frequency (8 to 12 Hz) in F4. Rettention.1: 48 hours after the training protocol, the test was taken from the subjects. The test included a single block of 20 attempts at dart throwing. In other words, a similar pre-test was performed. Under pressure test: 48 hours after the retention 1, subjects performed 20 attempts under stressed conditions to manipulate the level of cognitive anxiety. The method of social comparisons, threat evaluation, and financial rewards that leads to increased cognitive anxiety was used. Retention.2: At the end and after 48 hours of under pressure test, a retention 2 was performed. To data analyze descriptive statistics and Mixed ANOVA was used. The results of mixed ANOVA showed that the main effect of the test sessions was significant. In other words, the effects of training have been to improve performance and to reduce errors in all groups. In addition, the main effect of the group is significant. Therefore, the type of intervention had a different effect on the dart throwing performance, and the groups had different progress. Also, the interactive effect between the test sessions and the group was significant. Therefore, it can be concluded that the interaction of test sessions as well as the type of intervention on performance were effective. Results indicate the amount of conscious motor processing for neurofeedback training group decreased at post-test 1 and, under pressure test but this reduction was not observed in the control group. The dart throw points for neurofeedback training group and control group in the post-test 1 compare to per-test were enhanced, but only neurofeedback group be able preserve this increase in the under pressure test. This finding is consistent with past studies (Domingues et al., 2008; Gallicchio, Cooke, & Ring, 2016; Janelle et al., 2000; Zhu, Poolton, Wilson, Maxwell, & Masters, 2011). Studies have shown that the NFT can convert abnormal brain frequencies to normal frequencies. NFT can be used in many sports and exercises (Wilson, Peper, & Moss, 2006). Changes in the motor cortex map are accompanied by the motor learning that has been confirmed. On the other hand, the neurofeedback training leads to the enrichment of motor activity (Domingues et al., 2008). In the present study, the protocol emphasized the right hemisphere and led to asymmetry. The asymmetry is the definition of skilled athletes (Janelle et al., 2000). Therefore, the neurofeedback training accelerates the motor learning. This study indicates, there are influences among neurofeedback training, conscious motor processing, and athletic performance. In other words, the neurofeedback training by reducing the conscious motor processing leads to the desired motor performance and creates automatic sense in the athlete.

CONCLUSION

The results of mixed ANOVA showed that the main effect of the test sessions was significant. In other words, the effects of training have been to improve performance and to reduce errors in all groups. In addition, the main effect of the group is significant. Therefore, the type of intervention had a different effect on the dart throwing performance, and the groups had different progress. Also, the interactive effect between the test sessions and the group was significant. Therefore, it can be concluded that the interaction of test sessions as well as the type of intervention on performance were effective. Results indicate the amount of conscious motor processing for neurofeedback training group decreased at post-test 1 and, under pressure test but this reduction was not observed in the control group. The dart throw points for neurofeedback training group and control group in the post-test 1 compare to per-test were enhanced, but only neurofeedback group be able preserve this increase in the under pressure test. This finding is consistent with past studies (Domingues et al., 2008; Gallicchio, Cooke, & Ring, 2016; Janelle et al., 2000; Zhu, Poolton, Wilson, Maxwell, & Masters, 2011). Studies have shown that the NFT can convert abnormal brain frequencies to normal frequencies. NFT can be used in many sports and exercises (Wilson, Peper, & Moss, 2006). Changes in the motor cortex map are accompanied by the motor learning that has been confirmed. On the other hand, the neurofeedback training leads to the enrichment of motor activity (Domingues et al., 2008). In the present study, the protocol emphasized the right hemisphere and led to asymmetry. The asymmetry is the definition of skilled athletes (Janelle et al., 2000). Therefore, the neurofeedback training accelerates the motor learning. This study indicates, there are influences among neurofeedback training, conscious motor processing, and athletic performance. In other words, the neurofeedback training by reducing the conscious motor processing leads to the desired motor performance and creates automatic sense in the athlete.

REFERENCES

Domingues, C. A., Machado, S., Cavaleiro, E. G., Furtado, V., Cagy, M., Ribeiro, P., & Piedade, R. (2008). Alpha absolute power: motor learning of practical pistol shooting. *Arquivos de neuro-psiquiatria*, 66(2B), 336-340.
Gallicchio, G., Cooke, A., & Ring, C. (2016). Lower left temporal-frontal connectivity characterizes expert and accurate performance: High-

alpha T7-Fz connectivity as a marker of conscious processing during movement. *Sport, Exercise, and Performance Psychology*, 5(1), 14.

Janelle, C. M., Hillman, C. H., Apparies, R. J., Murray, N. P., Meili, L., Fallon, E. A., & Hatfield, B. D. (2000). Expertise differences in cortical activation and gaze behavior during rifle shooting. *Journal of Sport and Exercise Psychology*, 22(2), 167-182.

Vickers, J. N. (2007). *Perception, cognition, and decision training: The quiet eye in action: Human Kinetics.*

Wilson, V. E., Peper, E., & Moss, D. (2006). "The Mind Room" in Italian Soccer Training: *The Use of Biofeedback and Neurofeedback for Optimum Performance*. Biofeedback, 34(3).

Zhu, F., Poolton, J., Wilson, M., Maxwell, J., & Masters, R. (2011). Neural co-activation as a yardstick of implicit motor learning and the propensity for conscious control of movement. *Biological Psychology*, 87(1), 66-73.

In: Neurofeedback   ISBN: 978-1-53615-167-1
Editor: Michael C. Hellinger   © 2019 Nova Science Publishers, Inc.

Chapter 5

THE EFFECT OF NEUROFEEDBACK TRAINING ON SELF-TALK AND PERFORMANCE IN ELITE VOLLEYBALL PLAYERS

Ebrahim Norouzi[1],* and Fatemehsadat Hosseini[1]
[1]Department of Human Motor Behavior, Faculty of Physical Education and Sports, Urmia University, Urmia, Iran

ABSTRACT

The use of neurofeedback is growing rapidly in sport psychology and sport performance. In the present study, we aimed to investigate the effect of neurofeedback training on self-talk and motor performance of elite volleyball players. The participants consisted of 15 male elite volleyball players. The study was performed in three stages: pre-test, neurofeedback training, and post-test. Neurofeedback training consisted of 1) sensorimotor rhythm enhancement and 2) prevention training to the frequency of 12Hz at T3. Both at the beginning and at the end of the study, self-talk and service scores were measured. Data were analyzed with paired t-test as well as descriptive statistics. The data analysis

---

* Corresponding Author Email: eb.norouzi@urmia.ac.ir.

indicated that self-talk decreased in the group of elite players at the post-test. In addition, the service scores showed higher improvement for the group of elite players at the post test. The results of the present study indicate that neurofeedback training, inner self-talk (analysis of skill), and athletic performance are inter-related.

Keywords: sports psychology, neurofeedback, volleyball, athletes

INTRODUCTION

Achieving higher motor performance in sport requires a good state of mental condition, along with physical exercise. Quantifying the mental condition during coaching is often difficult; however with recent advancements in the field, such as using neurofeedback tools, it is possible to record and represent the neuronal brain activity of athletes (Casey, Yau, Barfoot & Callaway 2012). Based on this, it is recommended to use the practice pattern of cortical activity in order to improve motor performance (Casey et al. 2012; Cooke 2013). The important point here is, in order to improve the performance of athletes and reach optimum conditions, the athletes should practice the neurofeedback training willingly. This includes being in a non-thinking state which is an important part of the training. This non-thinking state can be detected via a specific frequency of electroencephalography (EEG) and can be given to the athletes as feedback during some sports, such as Golf hit (Vickers 2007). Research findings in the field show that, right-handed subjects the increase in alpha activity of the left hemisphere and the inhibition 12Hz frequency activities at T3 can be used as indicators of decreases in disruption and elimination of self-talking. Expert athletes show more cortex specific activities than novices during planning and implementing movements (Wilson, Peper & Moss 2006). For example, in expert athletes, reduced verbal-analytic in the left temporal region is pronounced. Therefore, neurofeedback training should be designed to increase the activity of sensorimotor rhythm (SMR) and reduce specific activity frequency of 12Hz at T3 to facilitate motor performance in the subjects.

METHODS

Participants

The participants of this study were chosen among the male volleyball players of Urmia municipality sport club team playing in the autumn of 2016. All participants were right handed (assessed by the Edinburgh Handedness Inventory) and had no previous experience in taking part in a neurofeedback training intervention. The average age of the participants was 23.8 ± 4.2 years old. The study was performed in three stages which were implemented consecutively without gaps: 1) pre-test phase; 2) neurofeedback training; 3) post-test phase.

Pre-test: During the first stage, after completing the questionnaire of evaluating the use of self-talk, 10 trials of standardized volleyball serve tests with the right hand were taken from each participant.

Neurofeedback training: this stage was administered immediately after the pre-test. In the present study neurofeedback training was performed as an independent variable using specific computer systems. The training took place in one session with the aim of increasing sensorimotor rhythm in each participant. After a 10-minute warm-up, participants were first asked to undergo an EEG recording. EEGs were recorded at 3 electrode sites (C3, C4 and T3) corresponding to the International 10-10 system. All sites were initially referenced to A1 to linked ears. EEG data were collected and amplified using a ProComp Infiniti with BioGraph software. EEG signals were sampled at 12-15Hz and recorded online. The electrode for SMR trainig was placed at C3 and C4 with the reference placed on the right ear. The signal was converted and the band filtered to extract the SMR (12-15Hz). The amplitude of the SMR was transformed online into graphical feedback representations including the audio-feedback tone by acoustic bass in the BioGraph software. Graphical feedback was provided in the form of pictures and games, for example a boat game . In this game, three boats appeared to the participant who was asked to steer the boat between two other boats to win. When the boat moveed it maintained the conditions above. In the SMR training the middle boat represented the SMR and the two other boats represented the delta and theta waves. When the particpants maintained SMR on theta and beta waves above the threshold 80% of the time, and maintained two theta and beta waves below the threshold 20% of the time, the middle boat began to move. Atthe beginning of training, participants had inhibitions 12Hz frequency in T3 (part of internal self-talk) to start SMR neurofeedback training. In other words, inhibitions 12Hz are necessary for entry into SMR neurofeedback training. Participants underwent a one-session training programme lasting one day. Each session of neurofeedback training lasting from 30 to 45 minutes. On average, training trials were performed in a single session . If the participants felt tired during training, short breaks were considered. The SMR NFT group aimed to increase absolute SMR amplitude over the designated threshold. The adjustment of the training difficulty threshold was employed to enhance the participants' efficacy during NFTprogressively.

Post-test:This stage was performed immediately after neurofeedback training. At this stage, similar to the pre-test stage, 10 trials of standardized volleyball serve tests with the dominant hand were taken from each participant. Additionally, they were asked to complete the questionnaire to evaluate of the use of self-talk.

CONCLUSION

The purpose of this study was to investigate the effect of sessions of neurofeedback training on the internal self-talk and motor performance in elite volleyball players. The results showed that the use of internal self-talk for elite (P=0.01) is significantly decreased in the post-test stage. In other words inhibition neurofeedback training decreased the amount of self-talk in the elite athletic group. This finding is consistent with results of Wilson et al. (2006). In this regard it can be stated that, neurofeedback training can be used in many sports and training and according to different protocol can be used to improve skills. As an example of neurofeedback training protocol that was used in this study, individual brain waves are used to change what is happening in plate on the monitor. For example, they use brain waves, for producing and doing games or sounds. The brain receives these activities as a gift and using this positive reward, brain selects constantly good waves eventually leads to permanent changes in brain function (Vickers 2007). In general, it can be stated that the inhibition of neurofeedback method reduces the self-talk and self-talk reduction associated with improved performance. However, this improvement was more because of reduced diversion of attention in elite. So, this kind of neurofeedback training protocol is recommended for expert athletic. In addition, the inhibition of self-talk method should be connected to the new coaching methods that ask athletes to prevent all the self-assessment.

REFERENCES

Casey, M., Yau, A., Barfoot, K., & Callaway, A. (2012). *Data mining of portable EEG brain wave signals for sports performance analysis: An Archery case study.*

Cooke, A. (2013). Readying the head and steadying the heart: a review of cortical and cardiac studies of preparation for action in sport. *International Review of Sport and Exercise Psychology, 6*(1), 122 - 138.

Vickers, J. N. (2007). *Perception, cognition, and decision training: The quiet eye in action*: Human Kinetics.

Wilson, V. E., Peper, E., & Moss, D. (2006). "The Mind Room" in Italian Soccer Training: The Use of Biofeedback and Neurofeedback for Optimum Performance. *Biofeedback, 34*(3).

In: Neurofeedback　　　　　　　ISBN: 978-1-53615-167-1
Editor: Michael C. Hellinger　　　© 2019 Nova Science Publishers, Inc.

Chapter 6

EFFECTS OF NEUROFEEDBACK TRAINING ON ALPHA POWER SUPPRESSION AND DART SKILL AMONG ELITE DARTS PLAYERS

Ebrahim Norouzi[1], Fatemeh Sadat Hosseini[1]
and Mohammad Vaezmosavi[2]
[1]Department of Human Motor Behavior, Faculty of Sport Sciences,
Urmia University, Urmia, Iran
[2]Department of Physical Education, Faculty of Social Sciences,
Emam Hossien University, Tehran, Iran

ABSTRACT

The aim of this study was to investigate the effect of Neurofeedback Training (NFT) on alpha power and performance of dart throw. A total of 20 elite dart players were randomly assigned either to the NFT, and a control condition. NFT consisted of training to achieve alpha-wave inhibition in F4, while participants in the control condition practiced dart playing with unrelated NFT. Dart playing skills and alpha were assessed four times: at baseline, 4 session later, under stress conditions, and at study end. Over time, alpha power and radial errors reduced, but more so in the NFT condition than in the control condition. Furthermore, performance in the NFT conditions also remained stable under stress. The results indicate that among elite dart players and compared to a control condition, NFT provide significant improvements in implicit motor skills. Importantly, dart performance under NFT conditions also remained stable under stress.

Keywords: elite players, alpha power, darts playing, non-thinking, neurofeedback

INTRODUCTION

Shooting sport such as dart is fine motor skill sport, that for success in this sport, high level of accuracy and grate motor control is required (Rienhoff, Baker, Fischer, Strauss, & Schorer, 2012). An important element in sport is athletes should be automatically to perform quickly and effectively. In other words, if task-relevant explicit (declarative) knowledge used in sport performance, the automatic motor control is disturbed (Gallicchio, Cooke, & Ring, 2016). Obviously, motor skill is learned through the passage from declarative knowledge to procedural knowledge. However, as results of training, learner enters the automatic stage. At automatic stage, skills are became implicit, and non-verbal (Lam, Maxwell, & Masters, 2009). These explanations are particularly true for sports such as sport shooting, and darts, in which concentration and excellent fine-motor skills are crucial to success and accuracy of performance (Rienhoff et al., 2012).

It has been confirmed that to dart victory, an optimum level of concentration and quiet movements are required. To summarize, it appears that in many sports reducing cognitive activity seems to benefit performance. In other words, optimal performance seems to be associated with a state of quiet mind (QM) (Wilson, Peper, & Moss, 2006). Previous research has shown that there are several ways to improve the implicit learning of motor skills. Here, we advocate one additional techniques, Neurofeedback Training (NFT).

The definition of Quiet mind is that for optimal performance, athletes should perform skills automatically (Wilson et al., 2006). This situation is also called a "non-thinking" and considered an important element of the sport performance. This unconscious state can be detected via a specific EEG frequency and presented as feedback to the athlete (Casey, Yau, Barfoot, & Callaway, 2012). One of the ways to achieve this state is reduced conscious control of performance.

METHODS

Participants

Twenty young elite dart players (mean age: M = 24.53 years, SD = 4.73) took part in the study. Inclusion criteria were 1) elite in dart skill; 2) aged between 19 years and 30 years, 3) willing to follow the study protocol and 4) signed written informed consent.

The present research method was Randomize Control Trial (RCT). Elite dart players were randomly assigned to one of two groups: 1) NFT, or 2) Control (mock neurofeedback). Next, participants were trained for 4 session according to the specific interventions. Their dart performance and EEG (Alpha power) were assessed four times: at baseline, 4 session later, under stress conditions, and at study end. They completed 200 dart throw attempts during training.

CONCLUSION

This study is the first to examine the effectiveness neurofeedback on motor performance enhancement. However, we also investigate alpha power after neurofeedback training. The key findings of the present study were that neurofeedback training impacted on both motor performance and alpha power in elite dart thrower. Moreover, compared to a control condition, neurofeedback training decreased alpha power and improved of dart throw performance. Interesting finding of present study is the maintained the motor performance of the neurofeedback training group in high-anxiety condition. The current study adds to the literature in showing that the motor performance of the neurofeedback training group was also sustained at a higher level under stress conditions. While the available data from the study cannot shed any direct light on the underlying neurophysiological and neuropsychological mechanisms, we propose that the following is a plausible interpretation. Alpha suppression resulted in automatic sense and leads to reduced conscious control of performance (Gallicchio, 2017). Implicit encoding in the learning process is a feature of skilled athlete (Wine et al., 2013) that can facilitate this process by using the neurofeedback training. Alpha as an EEG variable represents cognitive activity (Gallicchio, 2016, Zaidel, & Barnea, 2006). In line with Gardner and Moore's (2006), cognitive activity can be reduced by neurofeedback training. This method of reduces of conscious control of performance is associated with a new coaching approach that requires athletes to discourage self-assessment (Wilson et al., 2011). Based on the findings of Janelle et al, (2000), when alpha is reduced at F4, the use of visuo-spatial resources increased and leads to improve motor performance.

The limitation of the present study is not to investigate the effect of neurofeedback on non-skilled athletes, and the need for examine of this type of intervention is recommended to improve the performance of novice athletes in future research. Traditionally, there is a claim that increasing the alpha leads to reduced cortex activity (Hammond, 2007). However, based on the findings of Janelle et al. (2000), when alpha power at F4 is reduced the use of visuo-spatial resources increased and leads to improved motor performance. We therefore suggest that future research should consider changes in vision parameter following neurofeedback training. We also recommend that visual strategy variables such as visual fixation and quiet eye as a dependent variable should be examined.

REFERENCES

Casey, M., Yau, A., Barfoot, K., & Callaway, A. (2012). Data mining of portable EEG brain wave signals for sports performance analysis: *An Archery case study.*

Gallicchio, G., Cooke, A., & Ring, C. (2016). Lower left temporal-frontal connectivity characterizes expert and accurate performance: High-alpha T7-Fz connectivity as a marker of conscious processing during movement. *Sport, Exercise, and Performance Psychology,* 5(1), 14.

Lam, W. K., Maxwell, J. P., & Masters, R. S. (2009). Analogy versus explicit learning of a modified basketball shooting task: performance and kinematic outcomes. *J. Sports Sci.,* 27(2), 179-191. doi:10.1080/02640410802448764.

Rienhoff, R., Baker, J., Fischer, L., Strauss, B., & Schorer, J. (2012). Field of vision influences sensory-motor control of skilled and less-skilled dart players. *J. Sports Sci. Med.,* 11(3), 542-550.

Wilson, V. E., Peper, E., & Moss, D. (2006). "The Mind Room" in Italian Soccer Training: The Use of Biofeedback and Neurofeedback for Optimum Performance. *Biofeedback,* 34(3).

In: Neurofeedback　　　　　　ISBN: 978-1-53615-167-1
Editor: Michael C. Hellinger　　© 2019 Nova Science Publishers, Inc.

Chapter 7

EFFECTS OF THE LENGTH OF PREFRONTAL NEUROFEEDBACK TRAINING IN CHILDREN WITH AUTISM SPECTRUM DISORDER

Estate (Tato) M. Sokhadze[1,2,*], Manuel F. Casanova[1,2], Yao Wang[1], A. Tasman[1] and Desmond P. Kelly[3]
[1]University of Louisville, Louisville, KY, US
[2]University of South Carolina School of Medicine, Greenville, SC, US
[3]Department of Pediatrics, Greenville Health System, Greenville, SC, US

ABSTRACT

Neurofeedback training is a treatment modality of potential use for improving self-regulation skills in autism spectrum disorder (ASD). Multiple studies using neurofeedback to target symptoms of ASD have been made. These studies differ among themselves in the type of training (e.g., theta-to-beta ratio, coherence, etc.), topography (Cz or Pz), guidance by quantitative EEG (qEEG), and number of sessions (e.g., 20 vs. 30, etc.). In our study, we proposed that prefrontal neurofeedback

---

* Corresponding Author Email: sokhadze@greenvillemed.sc.edu.

training would be accompanied by changes in relative power of EEG bands (e.g., 40 Hz-centered gamma band) and ratios of individual bands (e.g., theta-to-beta ratio); with increased effectiveness at higher number of sessions (e.g., 12 vs. 18 vs. 24 sessions). Outcome measures included EEG and behavioral ratings by parents/caregivers. In the first pilot study on 8 children with ASD (~17.4 yrs.) we used a 12 session-long course of neurofeedback from the AFz site, while on the second study of 18 children (~13.2 yrs.) we administered 18 sessions of prefrontal neurofeedback training. In the third pilot study, presently underway, we administered 24 sessions of neurofeedback. The protocol used training for wide band EEG amplitude suppression ("InhibitAll") with simultaneous upregulation of the index of 40 Hz-centered gamma activity. QEEG analysis at the training site was completed for each session of neurofeedback in order to determine the relative power of the individual bands (theta, low and high beta, and gamma) and their ratios (e.g., theta-to-low beta) within and between sessions. In all three studies we analyzed Aberrant Behavior Checklist (ABC) ratings by caregivers (pre- and post-treatment). The pilot study that used 12 sessions showed only a trend of progress across the sessions even though changes of individual EEG bands and their ratios during individual sessions were significant. The 18 session-long course showed more significant improvements both in behavioral and prefrontal qEEG measures. We found a significant reduction in Lethargy/Social Withdrawal subscale of the ABC and decrease in Hyperactivity scores. In the 24 session-long study children with ASD (N = 6) were only partially analyzed as the study is still in progress and targets recruitment of at least 12 subjects. Our experiments showed advantages of 18 sessions-long weekly prefrontal neurofeedback course over the 12 session-long course. Children with ASD in a more extended neurofeedback course currently underway showed even more promising improvements in targeted neurofeedback measures and in behavioral symptoms of aberrant behavior such as irritability, lethargy/social withdrawal and hyperactivity. Future research is needed to assess qEEG changes at other topographies using brain mapping, more prolonged courses, and using other outcome measures including behavioral evaluations to judge the clinical utility of prefrontal neurofeedback in children with ASD. The current series support a need to address various factors affecting outcome of neurofeedback-based intervention, specifically the question of length of treatment.

Keywords: neurofeedback, autism spectrum disorder, EEG, aberrant behavior, gamma band

INTRODUCTION

Autism spectrum disorder (ASD) is characterized by severe disturbances in reciprocal social relations, varying degrees of language and communication difficulty, and restricted, repetitive and stereotyped behavioral patterns (APA, 2013). Standard treatment of ASD relies mostly on behavioral interventions (e.g., Applied Behavioral Analysis [ABA]) and pharmacotherapy for comorbid conditions such as anxiety, depression, etc. There is a need to develop and adopt neurotherapeutic approaches that will use applied psychophysiological training methods based on neuromodulation. One such technique is neurofeedback (NFB). This technique, a version of electroencephalogram (EEG) biofeedback, aims at acquiring self-regulation skills over certain brain activity patterns in an operant conditioning paradigm (Sherlin et al., 2011). By operant conditioning of EEG, NFB provides an effective way to train electrophysiological activity of the targeted cortical topography. Neurofeedback training is considered as one of the most effective and salient treatments for children with attention deficit/hyperactivity disorder (ADHD).

Clinical neurophysiological and psychophysiological studies showed that some EEG characteristics of ASD are similar to the reported brain EEG abnormalities in ADHD. It should be noted, that NFB is considered by several reviews as an efficacious and even specific treatment for some ADHD subtypes (e.g., inattentive type) (Arns et al., 2009; Sherlin et al., 2011). Neurofeedback training outcomes in ADHD symptom treatment were reported to be very positive and are well publicized (Arns et al., 2014; Sherlin et al., 2010). Currently there are controlled randomized clinical trials underway (e.g., design reviewed in Kerson et al., 2013) to further examine the utility of the method. This fact encouraged some research groups to apply protocols typically used in ADHD population in children with ASD, e.g., downregulation of theta-to-low beta ratio at Cz or FCz, upregulation of sensorimotor rhythm (SMR) at C3 or C4 topography with simultaneous downregulation of fronto-central theta rhythm).

The rationale for adopting the typical ADHD NFB protocols as an intervention of choice for ASD neurotherapy is based on the assumption that neurofeedback protocols successfully applied for treatment of ADHD may also be efficacious to the treatment of children with autism. The evidence that some of the symptoms of ASD can be improved with this approach has been reported in the literature (Jarusiewicz, 2002; Coben & Padolsky, 2007; Coben, 2008; Kouijzer et al., 2009ab). A study conducted by Jarusiewicz (2002) investigating the utility of neurofeedback in autistic children supports the proposition that the theta-to-beta neurofeedback training protocol, which is generally applied to ADHD, can also be of use in autism (Kouijzer et al., 2009b). However, according to Coben, protocols for ASD need to be selected and developed individually, since autism has a wide range of symptoms and variable EEG manifestations (Coben & Padolsky, 2007; Coben & Myers, 2010; Coben, 2013). Studies by Coben and his associates reported advantages of using qEEG-guided individualized protocols without limitation of treatment for enhancement/ suppression of specific rhythms or using the interventions which target only a pre-selected topography or is restricted to a specific EEG band (Nakatani et al., 2005; Coben & Padolsky, 2007; Coben et al., 2010; Coben & Myers, 2010; Coben, 2013).

Whether the current protocols that have proven efficacious in ADHD are also effective for ASD, or how to choose the appropriate protocols for core symptoms of ASD, are still open to questions. Such studies must eventually include analyses of the moderators and mediators of neurofeedback-based treatment process, biomarkers predicting intervention response, and should consider the mechanisms underlying learning of EEG self-regulation skills. The placebo controlled NFB studies should have well defined training targets, demonstrate ability to engage these targets, and show relevance of functional and behavioral outcomes to improvements in behavioral symptoms of autism. At the same time, there are multiple factors affecting neurofeedback treatment outcomes that require investigation before initiating a randomized clinical trial (RCT). Among such factors are the specific characteristics of the neurofeedback protocol (topography, selected EEG target, length of treatment, etc.) to be used as active treatment in the RCT. According to Arns et al., (2014) evaluation of neurofeedback for ADHD has gone through a long and winding road but still has to travel further in order to cover all grounds related to clinical effectivity and specificity. For the interested reader, we provide references to several published studies on neurofeedback training in autism (Coben, 2008, 2013; Coben et al., 2010, 2014; Datko et al., 2017; Friedrich et al., 2014, 2015; Hurt et al., 2014; Kouijzer et al., 2009ab, 2010; Linden & Gunkelman, 2013; Pineda et al., 2012, 2014ab; Sokhadze et al., 2014; Thompson et al., 2010; Wang et al., 2016; Zivoder et al., 2015).

Rationale for Prefrontal Neurofeedback for Gamma Upregulation

Our neurofeedback and qEEG studies were guided by experimental data and theoretical considerations related to specifics of high frequency EEG activity atypicality in children with autism spectrum disorder. Abnormalities of high frequency EEG oscillations have been associated with binding problems (the co-activation of neural assemblies) present in autism and other psychiatric conditions (Brock et al., 2002; Grice et al., 2001; Loring et al., 1985; Sheer, 1989). Oscillatory activity in the gamma-band of the EEG (i.e., 30-80 Hz) has been related to cognitive functions such as attention, learning, and memory (Kaiser, 2003). Binding of widely distributed cell assemblies by synchronization of their gamma frequency activity is thought to underlie cohesive stimulus representation in the human brain (Kahana, 2006). According to this assumption, changes in gamma EEG activity have been considered indicators of processing of Gestalt-like patterns (Herrmann & Mecklinger, 2000, 2001; von Stein et al., 1999). High frequency EEG oscillations in the gamma range, especially those centered around 40 Hz, are intimately related to mental processes such as consciousness (Llinas & Ribary, 1993), binding of sensory features into coherent percepts (Engel & Singer, 2001; Tallon-Baudry et al., 1996), object representation (Bertrand & Tallon-Baudry,

2000), attention (Fell et al., 2001), perception (Sedley & Cunningham, 2013), and memory (Herrmann et al., 2004).

There are only a few EEG studies employing resting-state examinations in individuals with ASD and practically all of them report oscillatory anomalies. Specifically, eyes open resting-state exams have shown greater relative delta and less relative alpha power in 4- to 12-year-old low functioning children with ASD (Cantor et al., 1986), and greater high beta and gamma power in 3- to 8-year-old boys with ASD (Orekhova et al., 2007). Eyes-closed exams have shown greater relative 3–6 Hz and 13–17 Hz power and less 9–10 Hz power in adults with ASD (Murias et al., 2007), and decreased delta and beta power, as well as increased theta power, in children with ASD (Coben, 2013). Although the aforementioned results implicate an atypical oscillatory activity in ASD, findings are discrepant and probably due to between-study differences in age, level of functioning, and medication status of the ASD participants.

Cornew et al., (2012) showed that children with ASD exhibited regionally specific elevations in delta, theta, alpha, and high frequency beta and gamma power, supporting an imbalance of neural excitation/inhibition as a neurobiological feature of ASD (Uzunova et al., 2016). In the auditory domain, reduced entrainment to auditory stimulation at 40 Hz in participants with ASD (Wilson et al., 2007) has been demonstrated. In contrast, during visual perception there is evidence for both hyperactivity and hypoactivity of gamma-band oscillations (Grice et al., 2001; Brown et al., 2005; Milne et al., 2009; Stroganova et al., 2012, 2015), raising the question of the link between high-frequency oscillations and perceptual dysfunctions in this disorder. Indeed, gamma-band abnormalities have been reported in many studies of autism spectrum disorders. Gamma-band activity is associated with perceptual and cognitive functions that are compromised in autism. Despite all of the evidence, the utility of gamma-band related variables as functional diagnostic biomarkers is currently unexplored, suggesting an urgent need for using gamma oscillation measures as targets of self-regulation training using neurofeedback as well as valuable and informative functional markers of response to interventions such as neurofeedback.

Neurofeedback of gamma frequency, specifically 40 Hz gamma was first explored in healthy subjects in a series of studies performed in late 70s and early 80s by a group of researchers headed by Sheer (Bird et al., 1978ab; Ford et al., 1980). Interest in using gamma activity as a target of neurofeedback-based self-regulation has been renewed during the last decade (Keizer et al., 2010ab, Kober et al., 2013, 2017; Sedley & Cunningham, 2013; Staufenbiel et al., 2014). Though some of these studies showed only moderate changes in gamma and less associated with improvements in cognitive functions as compared to other protocols, such as SMR training (Kober et al., 2013, 207), other studies did show improvements in cognitive functions and performance, as well as in improved memory retrieval (Keizier et al., 2010ab; Salari et al., 2014; Staufenbiel et al., 2014).

The series of pilot studies of our group addressed some technical, feasibility, acceptability, and conceptual issues need to be clarified to create pre-requisites for a double-blind randomized clinical trial of neurofeedback training for children with autism spectrum disorder. More specifically, in the series of studies we planned to develop methodology to monitor EEG activity and analyze changes during neurofeedback sessions in high-functioning children with ASD. The pilot studies represented one of the approaches aimed at the understanding of EEG correlates of neurofeedback training in high functioning ASD population, rather than an attempt at claiming clinical improvements resulting from the prefrontal brainwave training. Before moving to sham neurofeedback controlled trials it is proposed that more research studies should be done to understand: 1) whether children with high functioning autism can control EEG in NFB mode, 2) how EEG characteristics are changing during the training course in an ASD population, 3) what additional efforts are needed to correctly identify specific changes in EEG rhythms known to be abnormal in ASD, specifically gamma activity at the frontal sites, and 4) how many neurofeedback sessions are required to observe reliable changes in targeted neurofeedback indices and monitored EEG bands of interest. Another important factor is the specifics of neurofeedback protocol.

Our approach includes neurofeedback training at the prefrontal topography, specifically at the midline prefrontal site. Considering the role of the prefrontal cortex in executive functions, including attention and cognitive processes, it was feasible to investigate effects of neurofeedback using training at the anterior, frontal location rather than at the central or posterior (e.g., parietal) sites. This selection of cortical topography was also determined by our prior studies on gamma oscillations in children with autism (Baruth et al., 2010; Sokhadze et al., 2009) that showed alterations of evoked and induced gamma oscillations during attention tests especially well present at the frontal topographies.

The goal of this study was to conduct neurofeedback in children with ASD using the Peak Brain Happiness Trainer (PBHT, Neurotek, Goshen, USA) neurofeedback device with the "Focus/Neureka!" ("Focused Attention" index and "40 Hz-centered gamma" index) training protocol to investigate: relative changes in EEG bands (e.g., theta [4-8 Hz]) and sub-bands of interest (e.g., low beta [13-18 Hz], high beta [18-30 Hz]) and their ratios (e.g., theta-to-low beta, etc.) throughout the entire 12, 18 and 24 session long course of neurofeedback training in ASD, and during each individual training session. The aim was to investigate how 40 Hz centered gamma power and EEG bands ratios change during and between individual sessions within the course of neurofeedback training in high functioning individuals with ASD, and whether there are any correlations between EEG measures of interest (i.e., relative gamma power, theta-to-beta ratio) and neurofeedback training indices such as "Focused Attention" (i.e., "Focus") index and "40 Hz-centered gamma" (i.e., "40 Hz gamma") index.

It was expected that all participants would complete weekly sessions of ~25-30 min long training and learn to increase the "Focused Attention" index, and control level of "40 Hz centered gamma" parameter in neurofeedback mode. It was similarly expected that an increase in so-called "Focused Attention" measure of the PBHT device protocol would be manifested in a gradual decrease of theta-to-low beta and theta-to-beta EEG ratios, while an increase in the "40 Hz centered gamma" measure would be accompanied by the gradual increase of the relative power of gamma (35-45 Hz) band. We were also interested in exploring whether power of the selected EEG bands and their ratios correspond to and correlate with neurofeedback measures calculated in real-time on-line mode in BioExplorer-based commercial software application of the PBHT device.

The study explored our hypothesis that the relative power of gamma oscillations and the individual EEG band ratios will be changed and modulated as the predicted tendencies, in particular: (1) higher power of gamma during individual and across sessions; (2) lower theta-to-beta ratio during and across sessions; (3) positive correlation of the relative power of gamma band with the measure of "40 Hz centered gamma" index used as a neurofeedback training target, along with negative correlation of theta-to-beta ratio with a "Focused Attention" index measure which was also used as a target during the neurofeedback training in this study, and (4) the longer course of NFB training would have more profound effects showing acquisition of indices control, expressed as a gradual increase of target measures during and across the session.

METHODS

Patient Demographics and Recruitment

In the first of the series of pilot studies we recruited 8 children and adolescents with ASD diagnosis (mean age 14.2 years, SD = 4.7, 7 males, 1 female) and enrolled them in the 12 session-long course of neurofeedback training. In the second study there were eighteen children and adolescents (mean age 13.2 years, SD = 4.3, 14 males, 4 females) with ASD recruited. While in the third study, currently in progress, we recruited 8 (out of targeted 12) participants and report behavioral outcomes of neurofeedback in 6 subjects that already completed 24 sessions of neurofeedback training. In all three pilot studies (12, 18 and 24 session-long NFB courses) it was not required for participants to be off medication during the whole course of the neurofeedback trainings. We monitored medication status, dosage and other variables of pharmacotherapy and kept record, but were not used as a part of the patients' demographic descriptive characteristics in this study. Participants with ASD were recruited initially through the University of Louisville Weisskopf Child Evaluation Center (WCEC) (studies 1 and 2), and through Greenville Health System (GHS) Pediatrics Department (study 3).

All participants with ASD were diagnosed by experienced pediatricians according to the Diagnostic and Statistical Manual of Mental Disorders (DSM-IV-TR) (APA, 2000) or DSM-5 (APA, 2013) and further ascertained with the Autism Diagnostic Interview – Revised (ADI-R, Le Couteur, Lord, & Rutter, 2003) and/or ADOS/ADOS-2 (Lord & Rutter, 2005). Further medical estimations were made to exclude the participants with a history of seizure, significant hearing or visual impairment, a brain abnormality or an identified genetic disorder. Participants with severe psychiatric comorbidities were not included in the study. All patients were naive to neurofeedback training procedures and never participated in any previous neurofeedback study.

Using the Wechsler Intelligence Scale for Children (WISC-IV, Wechsler, 2004) or (for adolescents) the Wechsler Abbreviated Scale of Intelligence (WASI) (Wechsler, 1999), all participants were assessed to have full-scale IQ > 80. Child and adolescent psychiatrists and clinical psychologists at the WCEC and GHS performed pre- and post-neurofeedback clinical evaluations. Neurofeedback sessions were conducted by an experienced applied psychophysiologist certified in neurofeedback by the Biofeedback Certification International Alliance (BCIA). All required IRB-approved consent/assent forms were signed by the participants and their parents/guardians.

Behavioral Measures and Evaluations

In conjunction with the EEG data we collected the behavioral rating results with the pre- and post-neurofeedback data using the Aberrant Behavior Checklist (ABC) (Aman & Singh, 1994) from the parents of the ASD participants. *Irritability, Lethargy/Social Withdrawal, Stereotypy,*

Hyperactivity, and *Inappropriate Speech* were the five problem aspects that were contained in and assessed by the ABC rating scale. In our studies, we focused primarily on the *Hyperactivity, Lethargy/Social Withdrawal* and *Irritability* ratings before and after a course of NFB treatments.

Neurofeedback Protocol and Data Collection

In our pilot studies, ASD participants completed a course of NFB trainings using a "Focus/Neureka!" protocol designed to modulate the "Focused attention" index (FI) using "InhibitAll" type of protocol and "40 Hz-centered gamma" index (GI) using "Neureka!" protocol. The prefrontal neurofeedback training application used in this study was based on the BioExplorer software (CyberEvolution, Seattle, WA, USA) platform. The protocol provided the exercises for each subject to enhance FI and GI throughout the session while maintaining an adequate level of GI measure ("40 Hz gamma" index) within a certain range. During all of the treatment sessions different scenes from the BBC "Planet Earth" and "Life" series, as well as similar nature documentaries from National Geographic DVDs were shown to maintain the participants' interest. The protocol provided feedback to the subjects in both visual and auditory modalities. Based on the thresholds set, parameters related with visual feedback such as the brightness, size and continuation of the video have been modulated and the sound volume of the video adjusted simultaneously according to the targeted "FI" and "GI" indices during the treatment. All EEG signals and training parameters were measured using 3 electrodes, one active electrode at the prefrontal EEG (AFz) site, the second being a reference on the left ear, and a third sensor serving as ground and located between the two above electrodes. All of the subjects in the study were requested to complete a 25-30 minutes recording per session and a total of 12 weekly (study 1, N = 8), 18 weekly (study 2, N = 18) or 24 (study3, twice per week, N = 6 completed out of 8 recruited) neurofeedback sessions, in order to increase the "FI" and "GI" using the "Focus/Neureka!" Peak Brain

Happiness Trainer (PBHT) protocol. More than 90% of the sessions met the requirement of a 20-min minimum usable EEG data recording. Eye blink and EMG artifacts removal was implemented using the specific BioExplorer application that can be found in the operation manual of the NFB device.

The EEG Signal Processing

The EEG signal collected and recorded by BioExplorer applications during NFB treatments were exported using BioReviewer and further analyzed by a series of customized codes using Matlab software (MathWorks, Inc., Massachusetts). As an extension application of BioExplorer software, BioReview was used to export the raw EEG and to calculate the desired frequency bands of data for each session. By configurations in the BioReview report, along with the raw EEG, the separated delta (2-4 Hz), theta (4-8 Hz), alpha (8-13 Hz), low beta (13-18 Hz), high beta (18-30 Hz), and gamma (35-45 Hz) were also acquired using 7th order elliptical bandpass filters. The exported data were arranged in a text file in which the different items were organized into columns and each subsequent row represented the data point in time series between samples.

For the relative power calculation, it was necessary to gain the total power of the band from 2 Hz to 45Hz (the whole bands from delta to gamma frequencies). A custom band-pass filter application integrated of wavelet transformation and a Harris window configuration were created to filter and separate the 2-45 Hz frequency band from the raw signal that was exported from the BioReview reports. The wavelet analysis was used to provide enhanced temporal resolution of frequency responses of a given signal and it allowed us to apply a band pass filter to the individual waveform and avoid the distortion when applying the filter to the entire signal. Besides the relative power calculation for each band, the ratio of certain bands was also calculated. The ratios of interest for this study were theta (4-8 Hz) to low beta (13-18 Hz) – theta-to-low beta ratio, and cumulative theta-to-beta (13-30 Hz) ratio (theta-to-beta).

The primary statistical analyses in the study mainly included linear regression estimation and paired sample t-test methods. Each EEG dependent variable over 12, 18 or 24 sessions of neurofeedback course was analyzed using linear regression analysis. The mean values of pre- and post-NFB behavioral measures using ABC questionnaire were compared with the paired sample t-test method. EEG variables and FI and GI NFB training indices were calculated as well on per minute basis during each training session. Each dependent EEG variable went through the normality distribution analysis using t-test to ensure appropriateness for the test.

RESULTS

EEG Activity Measures Across Sessions of Neurofeedback

Study 1 (12 NFB Sessions)

Relative power of 40 Hz centered gamma activity (power within 35-45 Hz vs. total power in 2-45 Hz, in percentage) was found to show linear increase over 12 sessions of neurofeedback training ($R = 0.61$, $R^2 = 0.38$, $t = 2.45$, $p = 0.034$, power = 0.57 at $\alpha = 0.05$, lower than targeted level of 0.80). Theta-to-low beta ratio as well as theta-to-beta ratio did not show significant increase over 12 sessions of neurofeedback training in this study.

Study 2 (18 NFB Sessions)

Relative power of gamma activity showed a statistically significant linear increase over 18 sessions of neurofeedback (linear regression: $R = 0.49$, $R^2 = 0.24$, $t = 2.25$, $p = 0.039$, power of test 0.55 at $\alpha = 0.05$, below the desired level of 0.80). Theta-to-low beta ratio showed a statistically significant linear decrease over 18 sessions of neurofeedback ($R = 0.66$, $R^2 = 0.44$, $t = -3.57$, $p = 0.003$, power = 0.87). The ratio of theta-to-beta (i.e., theta ratio to sum of low and high beta, 13-30 Hz) showed a similar decreasing trend (t = -2.16, p = 0.045).

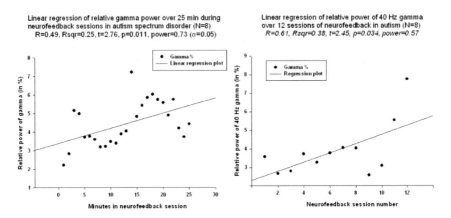

Figure 1. Left: Linear regression of relative power of EEG in 40 Hz range (35-45 Hz) over 25 min during neurofeedback sessions in 8 children with ASD enrolled in 12 session-long course. Right: Linear regression of 40 Hz-centered gamma power over 12 sessions of neurofeedback training in the group of 8 children with ASD.

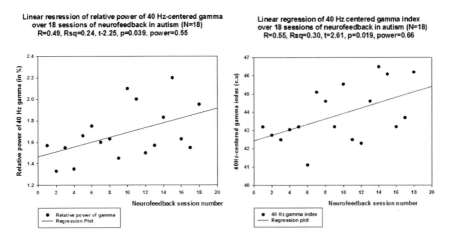

Figure 2. Left: Linear regression of relative power 40 Hz-centered gamma in 18 children with ASD enrolled in 18 session-long course of neurofeedback. Right: Linear regression of "40 Hz gamma" index over 18 sessions of neurofeedback training.

Study 3 (24 NFB Sessions)

Regression analysis is underway and will be reported when all 8 participants have complete the whole 24 session-long course, as of now only 6 subjects have completed the required number of training sessions.

Neurofeedback Training Indices

Study 1 (12 NFB Sessions)

The neurofeedback training measure of relative power of "40-Hz centered Gamma" index showed linear increase over 12 sessions of training ($R = 0.55$, $R^2 = 0.30$, $t = 2.61$, $p = 0.019$, power = 0.66). The "Focused Attention" index (FI) did not show a statistically significant linear trend towards increase over 12 sessions of the training.

Study 2 (18 NFB Sessions)

The "Focused Attention" index (FI, i.e., measure of "Inhibit All" protocol in neurofeedback) did not show a statistically significant linear increase over 18 sessions of training ($R = 0.42$, $R^2 = 0.18$, $t = 1.84$, $p = 0.084$, n.s.). However, the neurofeedback measure reflecting relative power of "40-Hz centered Gamma" index did show a linear increase trend over 18 sessions of training ($R = 0.55$, $R^2 = 0.30$, $t = 2.61$, $p = 0.019$, power = 0.66). Furthermore, this neurofeedback index showed a significant positive Pearson correlation coefficient with relative gamma power across 18 sessions of training ($r = 0.55$, $p = 0.019$). On the other hand, the "Focused Attention" index showed a negative correlation with the theta-to-low beta ratio ($r = -0.51$, $p = 0.03$) and with the theta-to-beta ratio ($r = -0.59$, $p = 0.01$) across 18 sessions of neurofeedback.

Figure 4 Illustrates changes of the "Focus" index in subject J001 across 24 sessions of neurofeedback and regression of the "40 Hz gamma" index in subject D002 across 24 sessions of neurofeedback training. Analysis of grand averages of all patients enrolled in the study is underway.

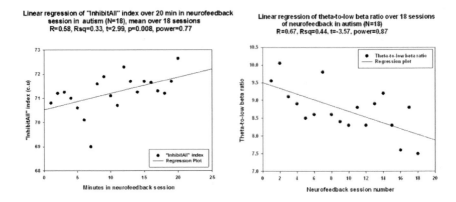

Figure 3. Left: Linear regression of the "Focus" index ("InhibitAll protocol) in 18 sessions of neurofeedback in 18 children with ASD. Right: Linear regression of theta-to-low beta ratio over 18 sessions of neurofeedback training in 18 children with ASD.

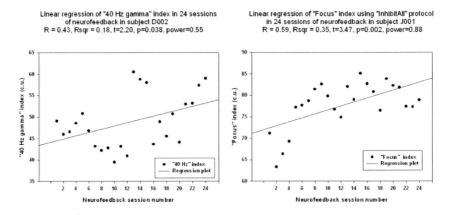

Figure 4. Left: Linear regression of "40 Hz gamma" index in a patient D002 enrolled in 24 session-long course of neurofeedback. Right: Linear regression of "Focus" index in a patient J001 enrolled in 24 session-long course of neurofeedback training.

Study 3 (24 NFB Sessions)

Analysis of FI and GI indices for 6 subjects in 24 session-long NFB course is in the progress and will be completed when all 8 participants will complete the study.

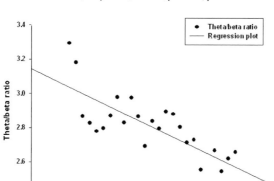

Figure 5. Linear regression of theta-to-beta ratio over 25 min of neurofeedback session in 12 session-long neurofeedback course in 8 children with ASD.

EEG Measures and Neurofeedback Training Indices during Individual Sessions

Study 1 (12 NFB Sessions)

Liner regression of relative gamma power (in %) showed statistically significant trend to increase over 25 minutes of neurofeedback training ($R = 0.49$, $R^2 = 0.25$, $t = 2.76$, $p = 0.011$, power = 0.73). Linear regression of low beta (13-18 Hz) was also increasing statistically over 25 min of training ($R = 0.53$, $R^2 = 0.28$, $t = 3.02$, $p = 0.006$, power = 0.79). Liner regression of theta-to-beta ratio showed statistically significant decrease ($R = 0.77$, $R^2 = 0.58$, $t = 5.73$, $p < 0.001$, with strong power=0.99).

Study 2 (18 NFB Sessions)

The "Focused Attention" index did show a statistically significant linear increase during each 20 min long neurofeedback session ($R = 0.57$, $R^2 = 0.33$, $t = 2.99$, $p = 0.008$, power = 0.77 at $\alpha = 0.05$). This index had a significant negative correlation with the theta-to-beta ratio during 20 min long neurofeedback sessions ($r = -0.70$, $p = 0.001$). It should be noted that the theta-to-low beta and theta-to-high beta ratios showed a high level positive correlation during training sessions (r = 0.63, p = 0.003).

Study 3 (24 NFB Sessions)

Analysis of relative power of 40 Hz gamma band and theta-to-beta ratio for 6 subjects in 24 session-long NFB course is in the progress and will be completed when all 8 participants will complete the study.

Behavioral Evaluations

Study 1 (12 NFB Sessions)

The only one statistically significant change in ABC scores was that for *Lethargy/Social Withdrawal* ratings that decreased from 5.88 ± 3.87 down to 4.25 ± 3.80, thus decreasing by only -1.62 ± 1.92, t(7) = 2.39, p = 0.048.

Study 2 (18 NFB Sessions)

There was a significant reduction in *Lethargy/Social Withdrawal* subscale of the ABC. The rating scores showed a reduction (from 10.18 ± 6.07 to 7.53 ± 5.82, change was -2.64 ± 3.13, t(17) = 3.29, p = 0.005), while *Hyperactivity* scores also showed decrease (from 16.65 ± 13.78 to 13.29 ± 11.97, -3.35 ± 5.39, t(17) = 2.56, p = 0.021). Correlation analysis showed that changes in *Lethargy/Social Withdrawal* scores showed a positive correlation with relative gamma power changes (r = 0.43, p = 0.041), and negative correlation with the theta/low beta (r = -0.43, p = 0.043) and theta/high beta ratios (r=-0.45, p = 0.033). *Hyperactivity* scores on ABC did not show any statistically significant correlation with EEG measures (i.e., theta/beta ratio, gamma) or NFB indices (i.e., "Focus" index, "40 Hz Gamma" index). *Irritability* rating showed a trend to decrease from 9.59 ± 7.65 to 8.17 ± 7.13, changing by -1.41 ± 4.33, t(17) = 1.35, p = 0.198, n.s.

Study 3 (24 NFB Sessions)

Irritability scores decreased from 15.00 ± 4.87 to 9.38 ± 3.63, -5.62 ± 5.99, t(5) = 2.62, p = 0.033. There was noted as well reduction in *Lethargy/Social Withdrawal* subscale scores of the ABC. In particular, the rating scores decreased from 10.18 ± 6.07 to 7.53 ± 5.82, -3.25 ± 3.73, t(5) = 2.46, p = 0.043. *Hyperactivity* scores decreased statistically significantly from 25.50 ±10.43 to 16.88 ± 9.12, -8.62 ± 8.33, t(5) = 2.91, p = 0.022).

DISCUSSION

The results indicate that the pilot study outcomes closely aligned to those predicted by our hypotheses, especially in regards to regression of the dependent variables across the neurofeedback training sessions. For instance, the theta-to-beta showed a decrement across NFB sessions in 2 studies while the relative power of the gamma band showed a linear increase over the course of the training in both 12 and 18 session-long courses. Both neurofeedback training indices ("Focused Attention" index and "40 Hz gamma" index) showed a linear increase over training sessions only in the 18 session-long course, as in 12 session-long study only relative gamma power increased significantly over the sessions. We found, however, significant trends of the EEG variables changes within the 20-25 min of individual neurofeedback sessions. Only one training index (i.e., "Focused Attention") showed a linear increase over the minutes within individual sessions in the 18 sessions study yielding a high negative correlation with both theta-to-low beta and theta-to-beta ratios in the EEG.

We found a notable decrease in the theta-to-low beta and theta-to-beta proportions from session to session in the 18 session-long course. These results are in accordance with the goals of NFB treatment described earlier for children with ADHD (Arns et al., 2009; Lofthouse et al., 2010). Even though the theta-to-low beta ratios used in prior ADHD NFB studies were mostly collected from the central or fronto-central cortical sites (e.g., Cz or FCz), our prefrontal theta-to-low beta and theta-to-beta ratios showed similar trends in an ADHD population (Hillard et al., 2012; Sokhadze et al., 2013). In this series of study, a reduction in the theta-to-beta proportions at the prefrontal site was robust across sessions only after 18 sessions of NFB treatment but not in a 12 session-long course.

Due to the improvements in behavioral outcomes indicated by ABC questionnaire, it is also possible to discuss whether training of the "Focus/40Hz gamma" measures of the PBHT protocol accompanied by the decrease of theta-to-beta ratio and increase of the relative power of 40 Hz-centered gamma activity are related to functional behavioral improvements reported by the patients. Determining which of these two measures is more fundamental to the effects of neurofeedback in ASD would increase the efficiency and aid in the delivery of more effective neurofeedback treatment methods.

As mentioned earlier, autism is characterized by an imbalanced inhibitory/excitatory ratio in local cortical network (reviewed in Uzunova et al., 2016), which may cause the disordered gamma oscillations in ASD reflected at the electroencephalographic level. The gamma abnormalities and excessive cortical excitation (E/I ratio) in autism have been considered as important EEG biomarkers for ASD based on recent theoretical reviews and experimental studies (Uzunova et al., 2016; Casanova et al., 2015). Brown et al. (2005) interpreted the abnormal gamma responses in their study on individuals with autism as reflecting decreased "signal to noise" ratio due to decreased inhibitory processing (Grice et al., 2001; Lansbergen et al., 2011). Brock et al. (2002) described the parallels between the psychological model of 'central coherence' (Frith & Happé, 1994) in information processing and their neuroscience model of neural integration or "temporal binding." This concept was further elaborated in an "impaired connectivity" hypothesis of autism which summarized theoretical and empirical advances in research implicating disordered connectivity in autism (Brown, 2005). The authors highlighted recent developments in the analysis of the temporal binding of information and the relevance of gamma activity to current models of structural and effective connectivity based on the balance between excitatory and inhibitory cortical activity (Belmonte & Yurgelun-Todd, 2003; Casanova et al., 2003, 2013; Rippon et al., 2007). Based on the minicolumn hypothesis of autism, disrupted patterns of coordinated high frequency oscillatory output in distributed networks might be associated with cortical "disconnection" in autism according to Casanova et al., (2006).

The current study indicated the potential of prefrontal neurofeedback aimed at modulating the disordered EEG activities associated with ASD. Also, from the results of the correlation between "40 Hz Gamma" index and the relative power of gamma calculated in our custom made program, the "Focus/40 Hz Gamma" protocol provided by the neurofeedback equipment used in our study can effectively help to improve gamma activity along with the decrement of theta-to-beta ratio in prefrontal EEG in children ASD.

Theta-to-beta ratios (both theta-to-low beta and theta-to-high beta) showed the significant linear decrease over 18 but not 12 sessions of neurofeedback. Theta-to-beta ratio is one of the classical indices for characterizing the ability to focus attention and to concentrate. The current study showed that both prefrontal theta-to- beta ratio and power of gamma activity could be modulated positively by operant conditioning during the NFB training in high functioning children with ASD. It is well known that most ASD subjects have difficulties with switching focused attention. The "Focus/40 Hz Gamma" protocol used in the study provided a successful way for positively modulating both gamma activity and focused concentration abilities in ASD. The positive effects of the neurofeedback training further can be manifested by the improvement in the behavioral scores measured by the ABC parental questionnaire. Our results show a significant reduction in the *Lethargy/Social Withdrawal* subscale of the ABC and a negative correlation with the theta-to-beta ratio. The *Hyperactivity* scores of ABC also showed a decrease (both in 18 and 24 sessions of NFB) but the same did not correlate with any EEG or NFB indices used in this study. The improvement of behavioral changes assessed by ABC before and after the 18 and 24 sessions of NFB treatments was in accordance to the functional outcomes seen in the EEG profile changes.

Our study showed that compared to previous protocols that required more sessions per subject (>30) and a more frequent training rate (e.g., twice per week), the statistical significant improvement either in EEG or in behavioral measures (Sokhadze et al., 2009) can also be achieved within a shorter number of sessions (i.e., 24 and 18 NFB sessions in ASD, or even 12 sessions in ADHD, Hillard et al., 2012) and weekly visits. Probably 24 sessions rather than 18 sessions might contribute to better consolidation of results of operant conditioning using neurofeedback, and currently we have studies in progress that will compare outcomes of 12 vs. 18 vs. 24 vs. 32 sessions of neurofeedback using the same protocol in children with autism. Our future efforts will be directed to combine the neurofeedback with other novel neuromodulation techniques employed in autism treatment (e.g., rTMS, tDCS, auditory integration training, etc.).

It should be noted that the study has several limitations. The enrollment to the neurofeedback training was open to only high-functioning children with autism, thus results cannot be directly interpolated for low functioning children with ASD. The study was not designed as a clinical research as it had no control group of participants, and the number of clinical behavioral evaluations was minimal. The focus of current study was directed towards more accurate analysis of the dynamic of target indices (FI and GI) and theta-to-beta ratio and relative power of 40 Hz gamma changes within and across neurofeedback sessions in children with ASD. Records of patients' demographic specifics (e.g., social status of families, ASD onset and duration data, etc.) and detail of their medication status were not analyzed. Analysis of some datasets for 24 session-long course was not complete, and is pending recruitment of a larger sample. In order to foster the neurofeedback treatment applications for children with ASD and its scientific rationale, further methodological advances are necessary: controlled and randomized study designs, larger sample sizes of patients, a more accurate selection of subjects with ASD, and more intensive and rigorous baseline, post-treatment- and follow-up evaluations.

Consideration of Important Factors during Designing Future Neurofeedback Studies

Recently papers have addressed important issues related to the use of neurofeedback, operant conditioning, and the role of learning (Coben & Ricca, 2015; Enriquez-Geppert et al., 2017; Gaume et al., 2016; Kerson et al., 2013; Niv, 2013; Pigott & Cannon, 2014; Pigott et al., 2018; Pineda et al., 2012; Ros et al., 2014; Sherlin et al., 2011; Strehl, 2014; Vollebregt et al., 2014; Zuberer et al., 2015). It is very important to have these papers reviewed and considered while developing neurotherapy protocols. Gaume et al., (2016) proposed that designing effective and efficient neurofeedback protocols would benefit from a comprehensive model of the mechanisms of learning during neurofeedback training procedures. Among the key elements relevant to such model, the authors listed perceptibility, autonomy mastery, and learnability. Within the framework of a proposed model, the number of neurofeedback sessions, duration of each session, time interval between sessions and several other related protocol details are crucial parameters of neurofeedback protocols. Ros et al., (2014) admitted that neurofeedback emerged as a promising technique that enables self-regulation of ongoing brain activity, but pointed out that despite empirical evidence of clinical benefits, a solid theoretical basis is still lacking on the mechanisms of NFB effects on these outcomes. The authors attempted to combine together several concepts from neurobiology, bioengineering, and theory of dynamic systems to put together a theoretical model aimed at describing mechanistic effects of neurofeedback training.

Strehl (2014) noted in her theoretical conceptual paper that even though the majority of definitions of NFB considers it as an operant conditioning method that results in acquisition of brain activity self-regulation skills, there should be considered beyond operant conditioning also role of classical Pavlov conditioning, two-process-theory as well as role of motivation in neurofeedback skills acquisition process. The model supports the hypothesis that learning aimed at self-regulation of EEG has to be considered within psychotherapeutic, or in other words within behavioral therapy framework. In behavioral therapy, the therapist assists patient to learn a new behavior focusing on overt behavior, cognition and emotions, while in neurofeedback therapist tries to help change the activity of the brain that becomes visible thanks to the biofeedback equipment. However, an important point is that therapist should know the rules of learning and be proficient in designing and applying neurofeedback training to be able to effectively guide patients in this version of behavioral therapy intervention (Strehl, 2014).

Zuberer et al., (2015) discussed role of the analysis of learning and adaptation processes during the course of training. The paper outlines the need to relate these processes to improvements in self-regulated EEG activity across training sessions to behavioral, neuropsychological and electrophysiological outcomes. At the same time, it proposed that more attention be devoted to the analysis of EEG changes and dynamics in the course of the neurofeedback training (both during the individual session and over the whole course of training) and how these measures impact on behavioral and clinical outcome. These suggestions call for the necessity of improving target analysis and monitoring EEG measures across sessions in the course of training and within individual session, assessment of learning trajectories in population under study, and to provide the best conditions for learning.

Pigott et al., (2018) critically reviewed the methodology from six sham-controlled trials using neurofeedback to treat ADHD and noted that some of the methodology may have violated established rules of operant conditioning by improperly using either automated or manually adjusted EEG reward thresholds. Some studies had as well other methodology flaws that may impede neurofeedback subjects from learning EEG self-regulation skills (Pigott et al., 2018). Some of such methodologically flawed studies led Thibault et al., (2018) to argue that these beneficial effects are due to placebo phenomena rather than specific clinical and behavioral effects of neurofeedback.

Discussions about NFB specificity should be encouraged to include analyses of the changes of targeted EEG parameters to be able to report learning curve, as well as changes of EEG measures in individual training session and across course (Zuberer et al., 2015). These changes should be correlated with the gains of behavioral and clinical outcome of the treatment course. It is necessary that for the evaluation of efficacy and specificity of NFB in autism strict methodological standards be adhered in the study design along with scientific rationale for the selection of the targets of EEG self-regulation. Several reviews and meta-studies (Coben, 2013; Hurt et al., 2014; Linden & Gunkelman, 2013, Pineda et al., 2014) have demonstrated the potential efficacy of NFB training with regard to the improvement of ASD symptoms. Whether NFB is efficacious and at the same time specific in neurotherapy of autism still needs further investigation and rigorous research, which should go beyond analyzing pre-post changes and must include analyses of the dynamic of targeted EEG indices and monitored EEG parameters during the process of EEG self-regulation skill acquisition.

CONCLUSION

In a series of studies with varying length of neurofeedback training sessions in children with ASD, we attempted to change the power of the gamma band and theta-to-beta ratio at midline prefrontal site to investigated whether these changes would influence behavioral symptoms. The results of our studies show that children with autism are indeed able to alter the power in the gamma band and theta-to-beta ratio if provided with neurofeedback. Our results also provide support for better expression of positive changes in behavioral rating scores following more extended length of neurofeedback course. Our results show that 40 Hz gamma index enhancing neurofeedback training increased prefrontal relative gamma power within sessions and prefrontal relative power of gamma across sessions both during 12 and 18 session long courses. At the same time, we showed decrease of theta-to-low beta and theta-to-beta ratios during session and across the course of neurofeedback even though "Focused Attention" index targeted by "InhibitAll" arm of the protocol did not show statistically significant increases. Neurofeedback had more profound effects on ratings of aberrant behavior following 18 and 24 sessions of self-regulation training. Results of these pilot studies will be used to inform design of the controlled trials aimed to evaluate clinical efficacy of the neurofeedback method in ASD.

ACKNOWLEDGMENTS

This study was partially supported by the GHS HSC Transformative Pilot Study Grant to Desmond Kelly.

REFERENCES

Aman, M. G., & Singh, N. N. (1994). *Aberrant behavior checklist - community. Supplementary manual.* East Aurora, NY: Slosson Educational Publications.

American Psychiatric Association (APA). (2000). *Diagnostic and statistical manual of mental disorders (DSM-IV), (4th ed.).* Washington, DC: American Psychiatric Association.

American Psychiatric Association (APA). (2013). *Diagnostic and statistical manual of mental disorders (DSM-5), (5th ed.).* Washington, DC: American Psychiatric Association.

Arns, M., Heinrich, H., & Strehl, U. (2014). Evaluation of neurofeedback in ADHD: The long and winding road. *Biological Psychology, 95,* 108-115.

Arns, M., de Ridder, S., Strehl, U., Breteler, M., & Coenen, A. (2009). Efficacy of neurofeedback treatment in ADHD: The effects on inattention, impulsivity and hyperactivity: A meta-analysis. *Clinical EEG and Neuroscience, 40*(3), 180-189.

Baruth, J. M., Casanova, M. F., El-Baz, A., Horrell, T., Mathai, G., Sears, L., & Sokhadze, E. (2010). Low-frequency repetitive transcranial magnetic stimulation modulates evoked-gamma frequency oscillations in autism spectrum disorders. *Journal of Neurotherapy, 14*(3), 179-194.

Belmonte, M. K. & Yurgelun-Todd, D. A. (2003). Functional anatomy of impaired selective attention and compensatory processing in autism. *Cognitive Brain Research,* 17, 651-664.

Bertrand, O., & Tallon-Baudry, C. (2000). Oscillatory gamma activity in humans: A possible role for object representation. *International Journal of Psychophysiology, 38*(3), 211-223.

Bird, B. L., Newton, F. A., Sheer, D. E., & Ford, M. (1978). Biofeedback training of 40-Hz EEG in humans. *Biofeedback and Self-Regulation, 3*(1), 1-11.

Bird, B. L., Newton, A. D., Sheer, E., & Ford, M. (1978). Behavioral and electroencephalographic correlates of 40 Hz EEG biofeedback training in humans. *Biofeedback and Self-Regulation, 3*(1), 13-28.

Brock, J., Brown, C. C., Boucher, J., & Rippon, G. (2002). The temporal binding deficit hypothesis of autism. *Development & Psychopathology, 14*(2), 209-224.

Brown, C., Gruber, T., Boucher, J., Rippon, G., & Brock, J. (2005). Gamma abnormalities during perception of illusory figures in autism. *Cortex, 41*(3), 364-376.

Brown, C. (2005). EEG in autism: Is there just too much going on in there? In M. F. Casanova (Ed.), *Recent developments in autism research,* (pp. 109-126). New York: Nova Science Publishers.

Cantor, D. S., Thatcher, R. W., Hrybyk, M., & Kaye, H. (1986). Computerized EEG analysis of autistic children. *Journal of Autism and Developmental Disorders,* 16(2), 169-187.

Casanova, M. F., Buxhoeveden, D., & Gomez, J. (2003). Disruption in the inhibitory architecture of the cell minicolumn: Implications for autism. *The Neuroscientist, 9*(6), 496-507.

Casanova, M. F., van Kooten, I. A., Switala, A. E., van Engeland, H., Heinsen, H., Steinbusch, H. W., Hof, P. R., Trippe, J., Stone, J., & Schmitz, C. (2006). Minicolumnar abnormalities in autism. *Acta Neuropathologica, 112*(3), 287-303.

Casanova, M. F., Baruth, J., El-Baz, A. S., Sokhadze, G. E., Hensley, M., & Sokhadze, E. M. (2013). Evoked and induced gamma- frequency oscillation in autism. In M. F. Casanova, A. S. El-Baz & J. S. Suri (Eds.), *Imaging the brain in autism*, (pp. 87-106). New York: Springer.

Casanova, M. F., Sokhadze, E., Opris, I., Wang, Y., & Li, X. (2015). Autism spectrum disorders: Linking neuropathological findings to treatment with transcranial magnetic stimulation. *Acta Pediatrica, 104*(4), 346-355.

Coben, R. (2013). Neurofeedback for autistic disorders: Emerging empirical evidence. In M. F. Casanova, A. S. El-Baz & J. Suri (Eds.), *Imaging the brain in autism*, (pp. 107-134). New York, NY: Springer.

Coben, R. (2008) Autistic spectrum disorder: A controlled study of EEG coherence training focused on social skills deficits. *Journal of Neurotherapy, 12*, 57-75.

Coben, R., & Padolsky, I. (2007). Assessment-guided neurofeedback for autistic spectrum disorder. *Journal of Neurotherapy, 11*(1), 5-23.

Coben, R., & Myers, T. E. (2010). The relative efficacy of connectivity guided and symptom based EEG biofeedback for autistic disorders. *Applied Psychophysiology and Biofeedback, 35*(1), 13-23.

Coben, R., & Ricca, R. (2015). EEG biofeedback for autism spectrum disorder: A commentary on Kouijzer et al., (2013). *Applied Psychophysiology and Biofeedback, 40*(1), 53-56.

Coben, R., Linden, M., & Myers, T. E. (2010). Neurofeedback for autistic spectrum disorder: A review of the literature. *Applied Psychophysiology and Biofeedback, 35*(1), 83-105.

Coben, R., Sherlin, L., Hudspeth, W. J., McKeon, K., & Ricca, R. (2014). Connectivity-guided EEG biofeedback for autism spectrum disorder: Evidence of neurophysiological changes. *NeuroRegulation, 1*(2), 109-130.

Cornew, L., Roberts, T. P., Blaskey, L., & Edgar, J. C. (2012). Resting-state oscillatory activity in autism spectrum disorders. *Journal of Autism and Developmental Disorders, 42*(9), 1884-1894.

Datko, M., Pineda, J. A., & Müller, R. A. (2017). Positive effects of neurofeedback on autism symptoms correlate with brain activation during imitation and observation. *European Journal of Neuroscience, 47*(6), 579-591.

Engel, A. K., & Singer, W. (2001). Temporal binding and the neural correlates of sensory awareness. *Trends in Cognitive Sciences, 5*(1), 16-25.

Enriquez-Geppert, S., Huster, R. J., & Herrmann, C. S. (2017). EEG-neurofeedback as a tool to modulate cognition and behavior: A review tutorial. *Frontiers in Human Neuroscience, 11*, 51. doi: 10.3389/fnhum.2017.00051.

Fell, J., Klaver, P., Lehnertx, K., Grunwald, T., Schaller, C., Elger, C. E., & Fernandez, G. (2001). Human memory formation is accompanied by rhinal-hippocampal coupling and decoupling. *Nature Neuroscience, 4*(12), 1259-1264.

Ford, M., Bird, B. L., Newton, F. A., & Sheer, D. E. (1980). Maintenance and generalization of 40-Hz EEG biofeedback effects. *Biofeedback and Self-Regulation, 5*(2), 193-205.

Friedrich, E. V., Suttie, N., Sivanathan, A., Lim, T., Louchart, S., & Pineda, J. A. (2014). Brain-computer interface game applications for combined neurofeedback and biofeedback treatment for children on the autism spectrum. *Frontiers in Neuroengineering, 7*, 21.

Friedrich, E. V., Sivanathan, A., Lim, T., Suttie, N., Louchart, S., Pillen, S., & Pineda, J. A. (2015). An effective neurofeedback intervention to improve social interactions in children with autism spectrum disorder. *Journal of Autism and Developmental Disorders, 45*(12), 4084-4100.

Frith, U. & Happé, F. (1994). Autism: Beyond "theory of mind". *Cognition, 50*(1-3), 115-132.

Gaume, A., Vialatte, A., Mora-Sánchez, A., Ramdani, C., & Vialatte, F. B. (2016). A psychoengineering paradigm for the neurocognitive mechanisms of biofeedback and neurofeedback. *Neuroscience and Biobehavioral Reviews, 68*, 891-910.

Grice, S. J., Spratling, M. W., Karmiloff-Smith, A., Halit, H., Csibra, G., de Haan, M., & Johnson, M. H. (2001). Disordered visual processing and oscillatory brain activity in autism and Williams syndrome. *NeuroReport, 12*(12), 2697-2700.

Herrmann, C. S., & Mecklinger, A. (2001). Gamma activity in human EEG is related to high-speed memory comparisons during object selective attention. *Visual Cognition, 8*(3-5), 593-608.

Herrman, C. S., & Mecklinger, A. (2000). Magnetoencephalographic responses to illusory figures: Early evoked gamma is affected by processing of stimulus features. *International Journal of Psychophysiology, 38*(3), 265-281.

Herrmann, C. S., Munk, M. H. J., & Engel, A. K. (2004). Cognitive functions of gamma-band activity: Memory match and utilization. *Trends in Cognitive Sciences, 8*(8), 347-355.

Hillard, B., El-Baz, A. S., Sears, L., Tasman, A., & Sokhadze, E. M. (2013). Neurofeedback training aimed to improve focused attention and alertness in children with ADHD: A study of relative power of EEG rhythms using custom-made software application. *Clinical EEG and Neuroscience, 44*(3), 193-202.

Hurt, E., Arnold, L. E., & Lofthouse, N. (2014). Quantitative EEG neurofeedback for the treatment of pediatric attention-deficit/hyperactivity disorder, autism spectrum disorders, learning disorders, and epilepsy. *Child and Adolescent Psychiatric Clinics of North America, 23*(3), 465-486.

Jarusiewicz, B. (2002). Efficacy of neurofeedback for children in the autistic spectrum. A pilot study. *Journal of Neurotherapy, 6*(4), 39-49.

Kahana, M. J. (2006). The cognitive correlates of human brain oscillations. *Journal Neuroscience, 26*(6), 1669-1672.

Kaiser, J. (2003). Induced gamma-band activity and human brain function. *The Neuroscientist, 9*(6), 475-484.

Keizer, A. W., Verschoor, M., Verment, R. S., & Hommel, B. (2010a). The effect of gamma enhancing neurofeedback on the control of feature bindings and intelligence measures. *International Journal of Psychophysiology, 75*(1), 25-32.

Keizer, A. W., Verment, R. S., & Hommel, B. (2010b). Enhancing cognitive control through neurofeedback: A role of gamma-band activity in managing episodic retrieval. *Neuroimage, 49*(4), 3404-3413.

Kerson, C., & Collaborative Neurofeedback Group (2013). A proposed multisite double-blind randomized clinical trial of neurofeedback for ADHD: Need, rationale, and strategy. *Journal of Attention Disorders, 17*(5), 420-436.

Kober, S. E., Witte, M., Neuper, C., & Wood, G. (2017). Evaluation of band, baseline, and cognitive specificity of sensorimotor rhythm- and gamma-based neurofeedback: Specific or nonspecific? *International Journal of Psychophysiology, 120*, 1-13.

Kober, S. E., Witte, M., Ninaus, M., Neuper, C., & Wood, G. (2013). Learning to modulate one's own brain activity: The effect of spontaneous mental strategies. *Frontiers in Human Neuroscience, 7*, 695.

Kouijzer, M., de Moor, J., Gerrits, B., Congedo, M., & van Schie, H. T. (2009a). Neurofeedback improves executive functioning in children with autism spectrum disorders. *Research in Autism Spectrum Disorders, 3*(1), 145-162.

Kouijzer, M. E. J., de Moor, J. M. H., Gerrits, B. J. L., Buitelaar, J. K., & van Schie, H. T. (2009b). Long-term effects of neurofeedback treatment in autism. *Research in Autism Spectrum Disorders, 3*, 496-501.

Kouijzer, M. E. J., Van Schie, H. T., De Moor, J. M. H., Gerrits, B. J. L., & Buitelaar, J. K. (2010). Neurofeedback treatment in autism. Preliminary findings in behavioral, cognitive, and neurophysiological functioning. *Research in Autism Spectrum Disorders, 4*, 386-389.

Lansbergen, M. M., Arns, M., van Dongen-Boomsma, M., Spronk, D., & Buitelaar, J. K. (2011). The increase in theta/beta ratio on resting-state EEG in boys with attention-deficit/ hyperactivity disorder in mediated by slow alpha peak frequency. *Progress in Neuropsychopharmacology and Biological Psychiatry, 35*, 47-52.

Le Couteur, A., Lord, C., & Rutter, M. (2003). *The autism diagnostic interview – revised (ADI-R).* Los Angeles, CA: Western Psychological Services.

Linden, M., & Gunkelman, J. (2013). QEEG-guided neurofeedback for autism: Clinical observations and outcomes. In M. F. Casanova, A. S.

El-Baz & J. S. Suri (Eds.), *Imaging the brain in autism,* (pp. 45-60). New York, NY: Springer.

Llinas, R., & Ribary, U. (1993). Coherent 40-Hz oscillation characterizes dream state in humans. *Proceedings of the National Academy of Sciences of the USA, 90*(5), 2078-2081.

Lofthouse, N., Arnold, L. E., & Hurt, E. (2010). A comment on Sherlin, Arns, Lubar, and Sokhadze. *Journal of Neurotherapy, 14,* 301-306.

Lord, K., & Rutter, M. (2005). *Autism diagnostic observation schedule, (2nd ed.).* Torrance, CA: WPS.

Loring, D. W., Sheer, D. E., & Largen, J. W. (1985). Forty Hertz EEG activity in dementia of the Alzheimer type and multi-infarct dementia. *Psychophysiology, 22*(1), 116-121.

Milne, E., Scope, A., Pascalis, O., Buckley, D., & Makeig, S. (2009). Independent component analysis reveals atypical electro-encephalographic activity during visual perception in individuals with autism. *Biological Psychiatry, 65*(1), 22-30.

Murias, M., Webb, S. J., Greenson, J., & Dawson, G. (2007). Resting state cortical connectivity reflected in EEG coherence in individuals with autism. *Biological Psychiatry, 62*(3), 270-273.

Nakatani, C., Ito, J., Nikolaev, A. R., Gong, P., & Leeuwen, C. V. (2005). Phase synchronization analysis of EEG during attentional blink. *Journal of Cognitive Neuroscience, 17*(12), 1969-1979.

Niv, S. (2013). Clinical efficacy and potential mechanisms of neurofeedback. *Personality and Individual Differences, 54*(6), 676-686.

Orekhova, E. V., Stroganova, T. A., Nygren, G., Tsetlin, M., Posikera, I., Gillberg, C., & Elam, M. (2007). Excess of high frequency electroencephalogram oscillations in boys with autism. *Biological Psychiatry, 62*(9), 1022-1029.

Pigott, H. E., & Cannon, R. (2014). Neurofeedback is the best available first-line treatment for ADHD: What is the evidence for this claim? *NeuroRegulation, 1*(1), 4-23.

Pigott, H. E., Cannon, R., & Trullinger, M. (2018). The fallacy of sham-controlled neurofeedback trials: A reply to Thibault and colleagues

(2018). *Journal of Attention Disorders*, https://doi.org/10.1177/108705 4718790802.

Pineda, J. A., Juavinett, A., & Datko, M. (2012). Self-regulation of brain oscillations as a treatment for aberrant brain connections in children with autism. *Medical Hypotheses, 79*(6), 790-798.

Pineda, J. A., Friedrich, E. V., & LaMarca, K. (2014a). Neurorehabilitation of social dysfunctions: A model-based neurofeedback approach for low and high-functioning autism. *Frontiers in Neuroengineering, 7,* 29.

Pineda, J. A., Carrasco, K., Datko, M., Pillen, S., & Schalles, M. (2014b). Neurofeedback training produces normalization in behavioural and electrophysiological measures of high-functioning autism. *Philosophical Transactions of the Royal Society of London. Series B, Biological Sciences, 369*(1644), 20130183.

Rippon, G., Brock, J., Brown, C., & Boucher, J. (2007). Disordered connectivity in the autistic brain: Challenges for the "new psychophysiology." *International Journal of Psychophysiology, 63*(2), 164-172.

Ros, T., J Baars, B., Lanius, R. A., & Vuilleumier, P. (2014). Tuning pathological brain oscillations with neurofeedback: A systems neuroscience framework. *Frontiers in Human Neuroscience, 8,* 1008.

Salari, N., Büchel, C., & Rose, M. (2014) Neurofeedback training of gamma band oscillations improves perceptual processing. *Experimental Brain Research.* 232(10), 3353-3361.

Sedley, W., & Cunningham, M. O. (2013). Do cortical gamma oscillations promote or suppress perception? An under-asked question with an over-assumed answer. *Frontiers in Human Neuroscience, 7,* 595.

Sheer, D. E. (1989). Focused arousal and the cognitive 40-Hz event-related potentials: differential diagnosis of Alzheimer's disease. *Progress in Clinical and Biological Research, 317,* 79-94.

Sherlin, L., Arns, M., Lubar, J., Heinrich, H., Kerson, C., Strehl, U., & Sterman, M. B. (2011). Neurofeedback and basic learning theory: Implications for research and practice. *Journal of Neurotherapy, 15*(4), 292-304.

Sokhadze, E., El-Baz, A., Baruth, J., Mathai, G., Sears, L., & Casanova, M. F. (2009). Effects of a low-frequency repetitive transcranial magnetic stimulation (rTMS) on gamma frequency oscillations and event-related potentials during processing of illusory figures in autism. *Journal of Autism and Developmental Disorders, 39*(4), 619-634.

Sokhadze, E. (2012). Peak performance training using prefrontal EEG biofeedback. *Biofeedback, 40*(1), 7-15.

Sokhadze, E. M., El-Baz, A. S., Tasman, A., Sears, L. L., Wang, Y., Lamina, E. V., & Casanova, M. F. (2014). Neuromodulation integrating rTMS and neurofeedback for the treatment of autism spectrum disorder: An exploratory study. *Applied Psychophysiology and Biofeedback, 39*(3-4), 237-257.

Staufenbiel, S. M., Brouwer, A. M., Keizer, A. W., & van Wouwe, N. C. (2014). Effect of beta and gamma neurofeedback on memory and intelligence in the elderly. *Biological Psychology, 95*, 74-85.

Strehl, U. (2014). What learning theories can teach us in designing neurofeedback treatments. *Frontiers in Human Neuroscience, 8*, 894.

Stroganova, T. A., Orekhova, E. V., Prokofyev, A. O., Tsetlin, M. M., Gratchev, V. V., Morozov, A. A., & Obukhov, Y. V. (2012). High-frequency oscillatory response to illusory contour in typically developing boys and boys with autism spectrum disorders. *Cortex, 48*(6), 701-717.

Stroganova, T. A., Butorina, A. V., Sysoeva, O. V., Prokofyev, A. O., Nikolaeva, A. Y., Tsetlin, M. M., & Orekova, E. V. (2015). Altered modulation of gamma oscillation frequency by speed of visual motion in children with autism spectrum disorders. *Journal of Neurodevelopmental Disorders, 7*(1), 21.

Tallon-Baudry, C., Bertrand, O., Delpuech, C., & Pernier, J. (1996). Stimulus specificity of phase-locked and non-phase-locked 40 Hz visual responses in human. *Journal of Neuroscience, 16*(13), 4240-4249.

Thibault, R. T., Lifshitz, M., & Raz, A. (2018). The climate of neurofeedback: Scientific rigour and the perils of ideology. *Brain, 141*(2):e11. doi: 10.1093/brain/awx330.

The rationale for using EEG biofeedback for clients with Asperger's syndrome. *Applied Psychophysiology and Biofeedback, 35*(1), 39-61.

Uzunova, G., Pallanti, S., & Hollander, E. (2016). Excitatory/inhibitory imbalance in autism spectrum disorders: Implications for interventions and therapeutics. *The World Journal Biological Psychiatry, 17*(3), 174-186.

Vollebregt, M. A., van Dongen-Boomsma, M., Slaats-Willemse, D., & Buitelaar, J. K. (2014). What future research should bring to help resolving the debate about the efficacy of EEG-neurofeedback in children with ADHD. *Frontiers in Human Neuroscience, 8*, 321.

Von Stein, A., Rappelsberger, P., Sarnthein, J., & Petsche, H. (1999). Synchronization between temporal and parietal cortex during multimodal object processing in man. *Cerebral Cortex, 9*(2), 137-150.

Wang, Y., Sokhadze, E. M., El-Baz, A. S., Li, X., Sears, L., Casanova, M. F., & Tasman, A. (2016). Relative power of specific EEG bands and their ratios during neurofeedback training in children with autism spectrum disorder. *Frontiers in Human Neuroscience, 9*, 723.

Wechsler, D. (1999). *Wechsler abbreviated scale of intelligence.* San Antonio, TX: Harcourt Assessment, Inc.

Wechsler, D. (2004). *Wechsler intelligence scale for children - fourth edition integrated (WISC-IV Integrated).* San Antonio, TX: Harcourt.

Wilson, T. W., Rojas, D. C., Reite, M. L., Teale, P. D., & Rogers, S. J. (2007). Children and adolescents with autism exhibit reduced MEG steady-state gamma responses. *Biological Psychiatry, 62*(3), 192-197.

Zivoder, I., Martic-Biocina, S., Kosic, A. V., & Bosak, J. (2015). Neurofeedback application in the treatment of autistic spectrum disorders (ASD). *Psychiatria Danubina, 27*(1), 391-394.

Zuberer, A., Brandeis, D., & Drechsler, R. (2015). Are treatment effects of neurofeedback training in children with ADHD related to the successful regulation of brain activity? A review on the learning of regulation of brain activity and a contribution to the discussion on specificity. *Frontiers in Human Neuroscience, 9*, 135.

BIOGRAPHICAL SKETCH

Estate M. Sokhadze, PhD

Affiliation: University of South Carolina School of Medicine-Greenville, Greenville, SC, USA

Education: MS in Biology, Tbilisi State University, Rep. Georgia, PhD, Institute of Physiology, Russian Academy of Medical Sciences, Novosibirsk, Russia

Research and Professional Experience: Psychophysiology, Neurofeedback, Biofeedback, Cognitive neuroscience, rTMS, EEG, ERP, Autonomic nervous system activity, Developmental disorders, Psychiatry and Behavioral Sciences

Professional Appointments:
- Research Professor, Department of Biomedical Sciences, University of South Carolina School of Medicine-Greenville, Greenville, SC, USA
- Gratis Associate Professor of Psychiatry, University of Louisville, Louisville, KY, USA
- Clinical Professor, Clemson University School of Health Sciences, Clemson, SC, USA

Honors:
- from 2014, President, Foundation for Neurofeedback and Neuromodulation Research (FNNR, ISNR Research Foundation)
- 2015 – Distinguished Scientist Award from Association for Applied Psychophysiology and Biofeedback (AAPB),
- 2009 – Joe Lubar Award for Advancement of Neurotherapy,
- 2018 – Ann-Marie and Joseph Horvat award for outstanding volunteer services (ISNR),

- 1998 - 2018 - Multiple citation papers awards from AAPB and ISNR (biofeedback societies).

Publications from the Last 3 Years:

Journals

1. Casanova, M. F., Sokhadze, E., Opris, I., Wang, Y., and Li, X.: Autism spectrum disorders: linking neuropathological findings to treatment with transcranial magnetic stimulation. *Acta Pediatr.* 104(4):346-355, 2015.

2. Li, J., Wang, Y., Yue, P., Liu, W., Yu, W., Ren, P., Sokhadze, E. M., Casanova, M. F., and Li, X.: Resting-state EEG relative power and functional connectivity in children with autism spectrum disorders. *Human Frontier Science Program* (HFSP) 9(1), 2015.

3. Sokhadze, E. M., Frederick, J., Wang, Y., Kong, M., El-Baz, A., Tasman, A., and Casanova, M. F.: Event-related potential (ERP) study of facial expression processing deficits in autism, *J. Communications Research*, 7(4):391-412, 2015.

4. Sokhadze, E. M., Tasman, A., Sokhadze, G., El-Baz, A. S., and Casanova, M. F.: Behavioral, cognitive, and motor preparation deficits in a visual cued spatial attention task in autism. *Appl. Psychophysiol. Biofeedback* 41:81-92, 2016.

5. Wang, Y., Hensley, M. K., Tasman, A., Sears, L., Casanova, M. F., and Sokhadze, E. M.: Heart rate variability and skin conductance during repetitive TMS course in children with autism. *Appl. Psychophysiol. Biofeedback* 41:47-60, 2016.

6. Wang, Y., Sokhadze, E. M., El-Baz, A. S., Li, X., Sears, L., Casanova, M. F., and Tasman, A.: Relative power of specific EEG bands and their ratios during neurofeedback training in children with autism spectrum disorder. *Front. Hum. Neurosci.* 9:723, 2016.

7. Sokhadze, E., Casanova, M., Tasman, M., and Brockett, S.: Electrophysiological and behavioral outcomes of Berard Auditory Integration Training (AIT) in children with autism spectrum disorder. *Appl. Psychophysiol. Biofeedback* 41(4):405-420, 2016.

8. Sokhadze, E. M., Casanova, M. F., El-Baez, A. S., Farag, H. E., Li, X., and Wang, Y.: TMS-based neuromodulation of evoked and induced gamma oscillations and event-related potentials in children with autism. *NeuroRegulation* 3(3):101-126, 2016.

9. Sokhadze, E., and Daniels, R.: Effects of prefrontal 40 Hz-centered EEG band neurofeedback on emotional state and cognitive functions in adolescents. *Adolescent Psychiatry*, 6(2):116-129, 2016.

10. Casanova, M. F., Casanova, E. L., and Sokhadze, E. M.: Leo Kanner, the anti-psychiatry movement and neurodiversity (Editorial). *Siberian Journal of Special Education* 1-2(16-17):6-9, 2016.

11. Sokhadze, E. M., Casanova, M. F., Casanova, E., Lamina, E., Kelly, D. P., and Khachidze, I.: Event-related potentials (ERP) in cognitive neuroscience research and application. *NeuroRegulation* 4(1): 14-27, 2017; http://dx.doi.org/10.15540/nr.4.1.14.

12. Sokhadze, G. E., Casanova, M. F., Kelly, D. P., Casanova, E. L., Russell, B., and Sokhadze, E. M.: Neuromodulation based on rTMS affects behavioral measures and autonomic nervous system activity in children with autism. *NeuroRegulation* 4(2):65-78, 2017.

13. Sokhadze, E. M., Casanova, M. F., Casanova, E., Kelly, D. P., Khachidze, I., Wang, Y., and Li, X.: Applications of ERPs in autism research and as functional outcomes of neuromodulation treatment. *Int J Med Biol Front.* 23(2):167-211, 2017.

14. Sokhadze, E. M., Lamina, E. V., Casanova, E. L., Kelly, D. P., Opris, I., Khachidze, I., and Casanova, M. F.: Atypical processing of novel distracters in a visual oddball task in autism spectrum disorder. *Behav. Sci.* 7(4):E79, 2017; http://dx.doi.org/10.3390/bs7040079.

15. Zeng, K., Kang, J., Ouyang, G., Li, J., Han, J., Wang, Y., Sokhadze, E. M., Casanova, M. F., and Li, X.: Disrupted brain network in children with autism spectrum disorder. *Sci. Rep.* 7(1):16253, 2017; http://dx.doi.org/10.1038/s41598-017-16440-z.

16. Kang, J., Cai, E., Han, J., Tong, Z., Li, X., Sokhadze, E. M., Casanova, M. F., Ouyang, G., and Li, X.: Transcranial direct current stimulation (tDCS) can modulate EEG complexity of children with autism spectrum disorder. *Front Neurosci.* 12:201, 2018; http://dx.doi.org/10.3389/fnins.2018.00201.

17. Sokhadze, E., ., Lamina, E., Casanova, E., Kelly, D. P., Opris, I., Tasman, A., & Casanova, M. F. Exploratory study of rTMS neuromodulation effects on electrocortical functional measures of performance in an oddball test and behavioral symptoms in autism. *Front Syst, Neurosci.*, 12:20, 2018.

18. Shtark, M. B., Kozlova, L., Bezmatenykh, D. D., Mel'nikov, M. Y., Savelov, A. A., & Sokhadze, E. Neuroimaging study of alpha and beta EEG effects on neural networks. *Applied Psychophys Biofeedback,* e-pub, June 11, 2018, https://doi.org/10.1007/s10484-018-9396-2.

Book chapters

1. Sokhadze, E. M., Frederick, J., Wang, Y., Kong, M., El-Baz, A. S., Tasman, A., and Casanova, M. F.: Event-related potential (ERP) study of facial expression processing deficits in autism. In: B. Flores (Ed.); *Emotional and Facial Expressions: Recognition, Developmental Differences and Social Importance.* NOVA Science Publishers, 2015, pp.109-130.

2. Sokhadze, E. M., Trudeau, D., Cannon, R., Bodenhamer-Davis, E., & Davis, R. E.: Substance use disorders and neurofeedback. In: M. Schwartz and F. Andrasik (Eds.); *Biofeedback: A Practitioner's Guide*, Fourth Edition, Guilford Press, 2016, pp. 707-716.

3. Sokhadze, E. M.: Lessons learned from Peniston's brainwave training protocol. In: A. Martins-Mourao and C. Kerson (Eds.); *Alpha Theta Training in the 21st Century: A Handbook for Clinicians and Practitioners FNNR,* BMed Press: San Francisco, CA, 2016, pp. 105-132.

4. Sokhadze, E., El-Baz, A., Tasman, A., Sokhadze, G., Farag, H., and Casanova, M. F.: Repetitive Transcranial Magnetic

Stimulations (rTMS) effects on evoked and induced gamma frequency EEG oscillations in autism spectrum disorder. In: M. F. Casanova, A. S. El-Baz and J. Suri (Eds.); *Autism Imaging and Devices*. Francis & Taylor Publ., 2016, pp. 497-536.

5.   Sokhadze, E. M., Casanova, M. F., Kelly, D. L., Sokhadze, G. E., Li, Y., Elmaghraby, A. S., and El-Baz, A. S.: Virtual reality with psychophysiological monitoring as an approach to evaluate emotional reactivity, social skills and joint attention in autism spectrum disorder. In: M. F. Casanova, A. S. El-Baz and J. Suri (Eds.); *Autism Imaging and Devices*. Francis & Taylor Publ., 2016, pp. 371-396.

6.   Sokhadze, E. M.; Casanova M. F.; Casanova, E.; Kelly, D. P.; Khachidze, I.; Wang, Y.; Li, X. Applications of ERPs in autism research and as functional outcomes of neuromodulation treatment. In: S. R Harris (Ed.); *Event-Related Potential (ERP): Methods, Outcomes and Research Insights*. Nova Science Publishers: NY, 2017, pp. 27-88; ISBN-10: 1536108057.

7.   Sokhadze, E. M.: Lessons learned from Peniston's brainwave training protocol. In: A. Martins-Mourao and C. Kerson (Eds.); *Alpha Theta Neurofeedback in the 21st Century: A Handbook for Clinicians and Practitioners*, Expanded 2nd edition. FNNR, BMed Press: Murfreesboro, TN, 2017, pp. 245-279; ISBN-9780997819434.

8.   Casanova, M. F., Opris, I., Sokhadze, E., and Casanova, E.: Systems theory, emergent properties, and the organization of the central nervous system. In: I. Opris and M. F. Casanova (Eds.); *The Physics of the Mind and Brain Disorders*. Springer International Publishing AG: Cham, Switzerland, 2018, pp.55-68. ISBN-10: 3319296728.

9.   Casanova, M. F., Casanova, E. L., and Sokhadze, E. M.: Dyslexia and autism: neuropathological differences pointing towards a spectrum of cognitive abilities. In *The Dyslexia Handbook* 2018. Penrose Group: London, 2018, pp. 63-70.

In: Neurofeedback   ISBN: 978-1-53615-167-1
Editor: Michael C. Hellinger   © 2019 Nova Science Publishers, Inc.

Chapter 8

MU RHYTHM IN THE IMPLEMENTATION OF THE BIMANUAL COORDINATION AMONG CHILDREN WITH AUTISM SPECTRUM DISORDER

Ebrahim Norouzi[1,], Fatemehsadat Hosseini[1], Mehran Solymani[2] and Sajad Parsai[3]*

[1]Department of Human Motor Behavior, Faculty of Physical Education and Sports, Urmia University, Urmia, Iran
[2]Department of Psychology, Faculty of Education and Psychology, Azerbaijan Shahid Madani University, Tabriz, Iran;
[3]Department of Human Motor Behavior, Faculty of Physical Education and Sports, Shahid Chamran University of Ahvaz, Ahvaz, Iran

ABSTRACT

Children with autism spectrum disorder have been sought to face the lack of motor control in their physical activities, however, some scientists stated that the reason for this weakness is dysfunction in the mirror neuron. In this causal-comparative study, the mu rhythm and bimanual

---

* Corresponding Author Email: eb.norouzi@urmia.ac.ir.

coordination was examined in 10 healthy, 10 high-functioning autism (HFA) in-active and 10 high- functioning autism (HFA) active boys. Participants performed bimanual in-phase and anti-phase movements with their wrists at two conditions including: 1) observation, and 2) execution, while EEG was recorded. Two-way mixed ANOVA was used to analyze differences between both outcome measures of HFA in-active vs. HFA active. Results indicated that HFA in-active and HFA active boys have higher mean of relative phase error ($P \leq 0.01$), moreover, have lower mean in mu suppression in both condition; observation ($P = 0.001$) and execution ($P = 0.001$). Results showed that a significant effect of condition for all groups. Findings confirm that HFA active boys performed bimanual coordination task more accurately. We have seen that when HFA boys perform bimanual coordination task, the mirror neuron activity has increased. These findings suggest that the special attention should be paid to motor activities in the treatment and the healing of HFA children.

Keywords: child, electroencephalography, autism spectrum disorder, functional laterality, motor skills disorders

INTRODUCTION

Autism is a complex disorder of mental development that seems to be a disorder of the nerve system that causes the dysfunction of the brain that is effective in causing autism (Deschrijver, 2016). Autism disorder (AD) characterized with abnormal social development, poor language capacity, difficulty in the imitation of others' actions. In addition, the damage in emotional communication and recognizing emotions is another important characteristic (Oberman et al., 2012). However, it seems that the collection of symptoms of autism is based on the functions of the mirror mechanism (Oberman et al., 2012; Perkins, Stokes, McGillivray, & Bittar, 2010). Therefore, the hypothesis is expressed that this collection of defects may depend on the damage of the mechanism of mirror neurons (MN) (Pascolo & Cattarinussi, 2012). The MN are a group of neurons in the cortex of the brain gray cells that exist in the regions of the brain including the premotor cortex, inferior parietal lobe, temporal lobe (Rizzolatti, 2005). MN is called key coordination elements due to its special role. MN has amazing power of effective mimicking the actions that will be observed involuntarily (Rizzolatti, 2005). MN show activity both during the individuals' performance and also when viewing the sensorimotor actions of others (Gangitano, Mottaghy, & Pascual-Leone, 2004). The function of MN makes the internal copy of the observed action that puts the observer in the position of an actor to imitate that action (Grèzes, Armony, Rowe, & Passingham, 2003). MN allow us to have direct domination on the minds of others and these dominations is not through the conceptual reasoning but it is through direct simulation and empathy (Carey, Perrett, & Oram, 1997). The theory of MN dysfunction in autism assumes that the behaviors of autistic children are due to serious damage to MN (Perkins et al., 2010). Therefore, it is guessed that the stability and the health of this MN mechanism, is the basis for the development of social skills such as imitation (Perkins et al., 2010). Anomalies in the early development of partial-frontal MN system cause defects in the autism spectrum disorder (Rizzolatti, 2005). Therefore, in order to improve cognitive function in these patients should be emphasized on the function of cortical neural systems, especially the function of MN (Perkins et al., 2010). The studies state that the interventions for treatment that the MN was targeted improved the functions such as imitation, social or even motor control in autistic patients. Therefore attending to MN in the autistic patients can be effective both in the diagnosis and in the treatment (Williams, Massaro, Peel, Bosseler, & Suddendorf, 2004). The Mu rhythm is a window that shows the activity of MN (Cheng et al., 2008). Mu suppression can be considered as a creditable indicator of the MN system activity (Pineda et al., 2008). When an individual performs an action or observes another person doing something, it leads to the reduction of Mu rhythm (Salmelin & Hari, 1994). Perkins et al. (Perkins et al., 2010) showed that in autism, the dysfunction of the MN can be seen. On the other hand, Mu rhythm is defined as an indicator of the functioning of MN (Oberman et al., 2012). Oberman et al. (2005) compared 14 autistic children with 14 normal children. The results showed that although those with autism showed an interruption in the Mu rhythm during voluntary movements, but this barrier was not seen when they observe the other person's movements (Oberman et al., 2005). An FMRI study has provided strong evidence to support the defects in the mirror mechanism in autistic children. While high-functioning autism (HFA) and normal children were to observe and imitate emotional state, brain imaging was carried out. The results showed that the activation in the frontal lobe was weaker in children with autism significantly compared to normal children. It is noteworthy that the degree of activation was correlated inversely with the severity of autism symptoms (Hamilton, Brindley, & Frith, 2007). Enticott et al. (2012) examined MN activity associated with social disorders in children with autism. The results showed that activity in the premotor/low anterior cingulate is significantly lower in autistic group compared to normal participants; that indicates the reduction of MN activity in this part of the brain in people with autism (Enticott et al., 2012). Cheng and et al. (2008) examined the gender differences in Mu rhythm which is an indicator of the activity of MN; they concluded that during the observation of the hand movements, women are stronger in the suppression of Mu rhythm than men. In this study just the motor acts were observed and examined and the performance of the motor task by participants was not considered. However it can be concluded based on the findings of this study that the subjects should not be examined regardless of their gender. In the present study, only the boys were used as subjects. The present study aims to investigate the rhythmic coordination movements in active and inactive autistic children. In previous studies, the reach-to-grasp movement (Grèzes et al., 2003) and gait deviations (Pauk, Zawadzka, Wasilewska, & Godlewski, 2017) are investigated and bimanual coordination movements have received less attention such as most actions that we do as activities of daily living, including coordination movements of the upper limb (Welsh, Almeida, & Lee, 2005).

Despite the studies mentioned above, few investigations were conducted about the broken MN in individuals with AD. Especially in this respect, slightly EEG studies have been conducted. Furthermore, Calvo et al. (Calvo-Merino, Glaser, Grèzes, Passingham, & Haggard, 2004) showed in a study that people who have higher skill levels than those with lower skill levels, more and stronger MN system activity occurs. Based on previously mentioned interpretations and investigations since these researches have not aimed to compare HFA active and in-active children, the aim of this study was to investigate this question; Is the Mu rhythm showing the activity of mirror neurons in two groups of children with HFA active and in-active different during observing and executing conditions?

METHODS

Participants

Participants in this study were boy's children with AD In the Iranian province of Urmia. Among the target population 20 patients were chosen. The participants were divided into two groups of 10 active and inactive HFA children. In addition, 10 healthy participants were selected as the control group. All participants were right handed (assessed by the Edinburgh Handedness Inventory) children and aged 6 to7 years with the age mean of 6.5 years. ASD diagnosis was conservative and based on DSM-I (Association, 2013) criteria, with positive scores on both ADOS (Lord et al., 2012) and clinical confirmation by child neurologist experienced in autism diagnosis (SHM). In other words, HFA participants were children with AD that did not damage their intellectual functioning (IQ> 75). The children were novices to the bimanual coordination task and unaware of the purpose of the study. The parents provided written informed-consent form, which has been approved by the local ethics board (Urmia University) before the start of the study.

CONCLUSION

The aim of this study was to investigate the Mu rhythm wave in implementation and observation of bimanual coordination task among active versus inactive children with HFA. The results showed that during execution in all groups and in all three regions C3, CZ, C4 Mu rhythm was active. Moreover, during observing the action performed by another person, region C3, CZ, C4 was active in all three groups, but not as much as the execution condition. In other words, the task performance increased activity of mirror neurons. Further, normal children compared to children with HFA, was stronger than the Mu suppression. This finding is consistent with Oberman et al (2005) study and Oberman et.al (2005) in a research that investigated the Mu rhythm in normal children and children with autism disorder. Their research results showed that the activation of mirror neurons significantly in children with autism spectrum disorder was weaker compared to normal children. In the present study EEG and motor behavior variables have been studied but the visual variables that were based on previous studies enhanced with improved function of mirror neurons (Oberman et al, 2013) were not considered. Therefore, it is suggested that future research will address the gaze behavior of subjects. In the present study the physiological factors that could have an influence on results controlled factors including age, hand dominance and similar education levels were controlled. However, in the present study, only children with HFA were used. It is suggested that, similar researches like the present study be conducted in female and with low function autism (LFA) children.

REFERENCES

Association, A. P. (2013). Diagnostic and statistical manual of mental disorders (DSM-5®): *American Psychiatric Pub.*

Calvo-Merino, B., Glaser, D. E., Grèzes, J., Passingham, R. E., & Haggard, P. (2004). Action observation and acquired motor skills: an FMRI study with expert dancers. *Cerebral cortex*, 15(8), 1243-1249.

Carey, D. P., Perrett, D. I., & Oram, M. W. (1997). Recognizing, understanding and reproducing action. *Handbook of neuropsychology*, 11, 111-130.

Cheng, Y., Lee, P.-L., Yang, C.-Y., Lin, C.-P., Hung, D., & Decety, J. (2008). Gender differences in the mu rhythm of the human mirror-neuron system. *PLoS ONE*, 3(5), e2113.

Deschrijver, E. (2016). *Self-other distinction based on motor and tactile processes in the autism spectrum*. Ghent University.

Enticott, P. G., Kennedy, H. A., Rinehart, N. J., Tonge, B. J., Bradshaw, J. L., Taffe, J. R., . . . Fitzgerald, P. B. (2012). Mirror neuron activity associated with social impairments but not age in autism spectrum disorder. *Biological psychiatry*, 71(5), 427-433.

Gangitano, M., Mottaghy, F. M., & Pascual-Leone, A. (2004). Modulation of premotor mirror neuron activity during observation of unpredictable grasping movements. *European Journal of Neuroscience*, 20(8), 2193-2202.

Grèzes, J., Armony, J. L., Rowe, J., & Passingham, R. E. (2003). Activations related to "mirror" and "canonical" neurones in the human brain: an fMRI study. *NeuroImage*, 18(4), 928-937.

Hamilton, A. F. d. C., Brindley, R. M., & Frith, U. (2007). Imitation and action understanding in autistic spectrum disorders: how valid is the hypothesis of a deficit in the mirror neuron system? *Neuropsychologia*, 45(8), 1859-1868.

Lord, C., Rutter, M., DiLavore, P., Risi, S., Gotham, K., & Bishop, S. (2012). Autism Diagnostic Observation Schedule. *Western Psychological Services*. Torrance, CA.

Oberman, L. M., Hubbard, E. M., McCleery, J. P., Altschuler, E. L., Ramachandran, V. S., & Pineda, J. A. (2005). EEG evidence for mirror neuron dysfunction in autism spectrum disorders. *Cognitive brain research*, 24(2), 190-198.

Oberman, L. M., McCleery, J. P., Hubbard, E. M., Bernier, R., Wiersema, J. R., Raymaekers, R., & Pineda, J. A. (2012). Developmental changes in mu suppression to observed and executed actions in autism spectrum disorders. *Social cognitive and affective neuroscience*, 8(3), 300-304.

Pascolo, P., & Cattarinussi, A. (2012). On the relationship between mouth opening and "broken mirror neurons" in autistic individuals. *Journal of Electromyography and Kinesiology*, 22(1), 98-102.

Pauk, J., Zawadzka, N., Wasilewska, A., & Godlewski, P. (2017). Gait Deviations in Children with Classic High-Functioning Autism and Low-Functioning Autism. *Journal of Mechanics in Medicine and Biology*, 17(03), 1750042.

Perkins, T., Stokes, M., McGillivray, J., & Bittar, R. (2010). Mirror neuron dysfunction in autism spectrum disorders. *Journal of clinical neuroscience*, 17(10), 1239-1243.

Pineda, J., Brang, D., Hecht, E., Edwards, L., Carey, S., Bacon, M., . . . Birnbaum, C. (2008). Positive behavioral and electrophysiological changes following neurofeedback training in children with autism. *Research in Autism Spectrum Disorders*, 2(3), 557-581.

Rizzolatti, G. (2005). The mirror neuron system and its function in humans. *Anatomy and embryology*, 210(5-6), 419-421.

Welsh, T. N., Almeida, Q. J., & Lee, T. D. (2005). The effect of postural stability and spatial orientation of the upper limbs on interlimb coordination. *Experimental Brain Research*, 161(3), 265-275.

Williams, J. H., Massaro, D. W., Peel, N. J., Bosseler, A., & Suddendorf, T. (2004). Visual–auditory integration during speech imitation in autism. *Research in developmental disabilities*, 25(6), 559-575.

INDEX

P

parenting, 31
parietal cortex, 111
parietal lobe, 118
participants, x, xi, 38, 39, 44, 45, 59, 61, 65, 67, 71, 73, 82, 84, 85, 86, 87, 91, 92, 94, 98, 120, 121
patients with impaired motor performance, 55
Peniston protocol, 19, 27
perceptual processing, 109
personal qualities, 5
personality disorder, 6
pharmacotherapy, 79, 85
physical exercise, 66
pilot study, xi, 31, 32, 33, 78, 95, 106
placebo, 5, 39, 50, 80, 100
positive correlation, 85, 94
positive emotions, 21
positive feedback, 38
post traumatic stress disorder (PTSD), 14, 32, 51
prefrontal cortex, 84
problem behavior, 12, 13
problem drinking, 30
procedural knowledge, 72
processing deficits, 113, 115
psychiatric institution, 40
psychiatry, 114, 123
psychological issues, 54
psychological processes, 48
psychology, x, 65, 66
psychopathology, 2, 6
psychostimulants, 33
psychotherapy, 4, 6, 7, 17, 19, 34

Q

questionnaire, 67, 68, 89, 96, 97
quiet mind (QM), viii, 60, 72

R

rating scale, 20, 87
reaction time, vii, ix, 53, 54, 56
real time functional magnetic resonance tomography neurofeedback (rtfMRT-NF), 39
recidivism, 27, 29, 30, 31, 32
reconstruction, 49
regression, 89, 90, 91, 92, 93, 95
regression analysis, 89
rehabilitation, 3, 54, 56, 57
rehabilitation program, 3
relaxation, 3
rhythm, viii, x, xii, 3, 65, 66, 67, 79, 107, 117, 119, 121, 123
right hemisphere, 62

S

schizophrenia, 6, 15
Scott and Kaiser modifications, 19
seizure, 86
selective attention, 103, 106
self-control, 9
self-regulation, xi, 48, 51, 77, 79, 80, 82, 83, 99, 100, 101, 102
sensation, 56
sensor, 87
sensorimotor cortex, 55
sensorimotor rhythm (SMR), x, 20, 55, 65, 66, 67, 79, 83, 107
sexual offending, 33
sexual violence, 12
sexually abusive behavior, vii, ix, 1
sham, ix, 5, 38, 44, 45, 49, 50, 83, 100, 108
shooting sport, 72
simulation, 38, 43, 119
simultaneous multiple sources (SMS-) LORETA, 41, 42, 44, 50
skill acquisition, 101

CRIME AND CRIMINAL BEHAVIOR

EDITOR: Analise Klein

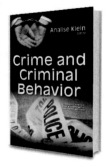

SERIES: Criminal Justice, Law Enforcement and Corrections

BOOK DESCRIPTION: In this book, Chapter One begins with a discussion on the use of dogs in the courtroom. Chapter Two explores the research on the criminal narratives of general offending populations, and introduces new insight into Mentally Disordered Offenders (MDOs), and the impact various mental disorders may have on the structure of criminal narratives.

SOFTCOVER ISBN: 978-1-63485-566-2
RETAIL PRICE: $95

NEUROLOGICAL DISORDERS: NEW RESEARCH

EDITORS: Chloe E. Thomas and Jayden R. Moore

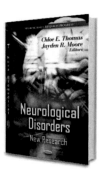

SERIES: Neuroscience Research Progress

BOOK DESCRIPTION: In this book, the authors present current research in the study of neurological disorders including advanced structural and functional MRI techniques used in Parkinson's disease and the role of neuropoietic cytokines in neural injury.

HARDCOVER ISBN: 978-1-62257-042-3
RETAIL PRICE: $145

DOMESTIC VIOLENCE: PREVALENCE, RISK FACTORS AND PERSPECTIVES

EDITOR: Mitchell Ortiz

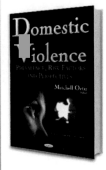

SERIES: Family Issues in the 21st Century

BOOK DESCRIPTION: This book provides an overview of the prevalence, risk factors and several perspectives of domestic violence.

HARDCOVER ISBN: 978-1-63485-795-6
RETAIL PRICE: $230

SEXUAL ASSAULT: PREVALENCE, HEALTH EFFECTS AND COPING STRATEGIES

EDITOR: Sheila Miller

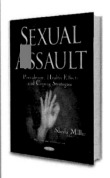

SERIES: Bullying and Victimization

BOOK DESCRIPTION: This book provides new research on the prevalence, health effects and coping strategies of sexual assault.

SOFTCOVER ISBN: 978-1-53610-514-8
RETAIL PRICE: S82